THRIVE
BEYOND TRAUMAS

A Guide for Trauma Workers and their Managers

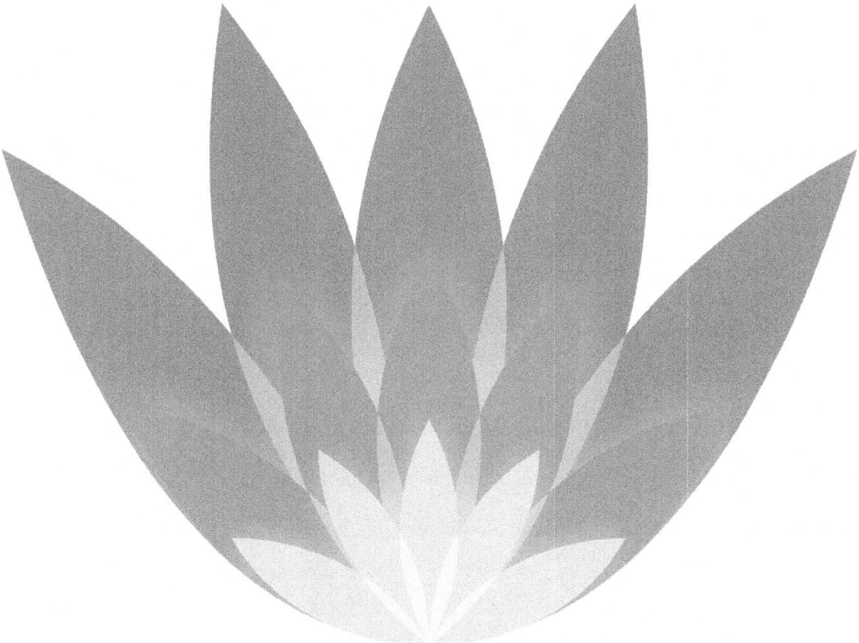

Margaret Bennett

First published in 2015

A Cataloguing-in-Publication record is available from the National Library of Australia.

ISBN: 9780994311634 (pbk.)

Disclaimer
All information in this book is for general use only. The general advice in this book should not be used as a substitute for advice from a qualified health professional such as a general practitioner or psychologist. The author is not responsible for any specific health or mental needs that may require medical supervision and is not liable for any damages or negative consequences arising from any treatment, action, application, or preparation to any person reading or following the information in this book. References are provided for informational purposes only and do not constitute endorsement of any other sources.

Printed by The OMNE Group www.omne.com.au

ACKNOWLEDGEMENTS

I wish to thank all my past and present colleagues, and my past and present clients, for inspiring insights I have gleaned over the years. You have helped me put my thoughts together, resulting in this book. Every organisation I have worked in has taught me something about how trauma workers fare in their workplaces; they can either become more inspired, or they can become so emotionally depleted that they subsequently have to leave their jobs to retain their sanity - and their life.

Even with the above support there are also special friends and colleagues who deserve special mention: Joan Whitely, Sue Beecher, Dr Sue Boyd, Dr Cecily Moreton, Leslie McLean, and Nancy Davis who keep me inspired and cheer for me. Then there are the members of my KPI accountability groups: Alex Allwood, Claire Broad, Anne Farrell, Alexis Hill, Karen Koedding, Jo Lia, Jacinta O'Connell, Robin Powis, Gabriela Rosa, Karen Sander, Victoria Tulloch, and Vanessa Varrto who kept reminding me I could do this; and of course to the KPI inspirers Glen Carlson, David Dugan, and Andrew Griffiths.

Special acknowledgements too go to my children who bring me back to earth when needed.

Thank you all for inspiring me.

Margi

CONTENTS

PRELUDE

As I begin to write this book about trauma workers and trauma, I am waiting at a specialist teaching hospital with a friend. Her medical specialist had emailed her asking her to come in to see him at short notice to get some results. He asked her to have someone with her. She suspects it is bad news.

Several months ago, an ex-lover I had re-established a relationship with after thirteen years (and significant 'torch-carrying' on both our parts) planned to come to Australia to live with me. Two days after confirming plans, he was hospitalised in another country and died a few days later (though he lovingly managed a phone call to me before he died).

I write these seemingly unrelated events as a reminder that we all experience trauma in our lives; it is a reality of life. Rare is the person who doesn't experience trauma. We give birth, we miscarry (for me five times), we lose children, we lose jobs, we divorce, we have accidents, and we lose friends and family in unforeseen circumstances. We live through all these experiences and sometimes more, and generally the longer we live the more likely we are to experience such traumas. While millions of people face these events every day, this book is for a particular group of people: trauma workers.

Trauma workers will have the same life experiences as many other people. However, what stands them apart is that they experience these events personally while working closely with people who have survived traumatic experiences themselves or while witnessing people in traumatic situations. So who are these trauma workers? They may be people who have chosen to work in fields related to trauma: doctors, nurses, social workers, psychologists, lawyers, welfare workers, ambulance drivers, and journalists to name but a few. Some of their training and career development mean they might have some knowledge of dealing with trauma in others. But are they immune to the effects of dealing with it themselves?

Trauma workers may also be people who have 'fallen into it' such as volunteers, supporters, and social activists. People who apply for jobs then witness events they had neither anticipated nor encountered before and which shocks them - such as working in a refugee camp.

These are regular people in a particular place at a particular time. For example, an ordinary day is shattered by a bomb blast for those watching the Boston Marathon. People travelling in countries when social unrest breaks out or natural disasters hit such as the earthquakes in Japan, or the tsunami in Aceh and Sri Lanka, or the mud slide in Scotland many years ago and more recently in Indonesia. These are situations where life changes in a heartbeat. What happens for these people?

This book addresses a few central questions shared by many of these people. *'How can my life go back to normal after witnessing or working in highly stressed settings that most people don't experience and may not be able to talk about? How do I manage to get through my own life's traumatic experiences while helping others through theirs? How do I go beyond my own trauma to thrive despite the work I do?'*

Chapter 1

So what do you know about trauma?

This question is often asked of me. Imagine the scene: it is a weekend and I am at a party. 'So, what do you do?' asks someone. Making light conversation or wanting to get to know me? I don't know. Does it matter? I pause for a second, 'Oh, I work with people,' I might say, or I dive in and say, 'I'm a therapist' (that either piques their interest or has them running away) or, 'I work with rape and domestic violence/child sexual abuse cases.' 'That must be hard,' they say or, 'how did you get into that?' and invariably at some point they ask, 'so what do you know about trauma?'

In answer to 'that must be hard,' I may say (not too flippantly I hope) 'oh not as hard as torture and trauma, or missing persons.' The other times I am asked that question is by clients. Their situation is that they have lost someone to cancer/they have a missing child/they have been brutalised at home and/or in the work place; and sometimes I do ask myself as well... what do I know? Not that I am suggesting that trauma workers need to have shared that experience with their clients, but many have.

This book is written for a specific group of trauma workers: those who have experienced trauma themselves or who experience it in the course of their work with trauma survivors. Some of the questions they may have are:

- What does it mean to work in a traumatic and traumatising environment?
- How do people become involved in trauma work?
- What is trauma and how does it affect people?
- How do you manage when you have little support in your work and/or life?

- How do you stay focused when you experience personal traumas in your own life while working with trauma survivors?
- How do you manage the inter-disciplinary issues that can happen in trauma organisations?
- How can your manager support you, and importantly;
- How do you thrive as a trauma worker and build a life after your time as a trauma worker is over.

I have been a social worker for over 30 years. My career has seen me take on roles such as group worker, workshop designer and facilitator, psychotherapist, family therapist, couples' counselor, sex therapist, team leader, health service manager, executive director of health and trauma services, academic in medical and social work faculties, trauma service evaluation expert, trauma consultant, and clinical and group work supervisor.

I have worked in small and large trauma services in major cities and country areas, and I have sat in remote camps with indigenous people in Australia and other parts of Asia hearing stories about how people survive their traumas and their work. I have won international awards for my work and am especially grateful to the Churchill Fellowship Foundation in Australia that allowed me to see how my work in establishing trauma services compared internationally.

I have been featured in newspaper articles and on radio and TV interviews, making the general public aware of torture and trauma, refugees, the need for accommodation services, the need for child care services in areas where there are none, or what prostate cancer does to men and their families and communities.

Although I have often needed to handle the prurient interest of those interviewing rather than their commitment to issues, I have also been blessed by being able to raise issues with accomplished and respected media commentators. Through all this I have learned that, like trauma survivors themselves, workers who know trauma from the inside out are a resourceful and resilient group of people who are all too often under-recognised in the organisations for which they work.

What is a trauma worker?

Many trauma industries have developed due to the gamut of human problems we all share. Trauma workers can be ambulance workers who see a child the same age as their own killed in a car accident; nurses who witness horrific deaths or deformities; volunteers who help out in emergencies after floods, bushfires, and earthquakes; nuns, priests and clerics who make their services available voluntarily; and counsellors who specialise in trauma theory after working with people with whom they share a traumatic experience.

A trauma worker can be a skilled and trained professional or an ordinary person doing something for others.

Many trauma workers work in isolation facing not only their work with challenging clients, but they may also witness trauma in their workplaces or in their homes: terminal illnesses, assaults, and deaths know no boundaries. While most work places have policies to provide short term support, the daily act of turning up to work and doing their job can be even more demanding physically and psychologically when they are working with trauma victims or survivors as well.

Early career professionals, that are people with less than five years' experience, may work with some of the most traumatised clients in areas such as child protection, rape, domestic violence, intimate partner abuse, and hospital cancer wards. Longer career professionals may become concerned they are becoming distant and jaded or, even worse, leave the trauma field completely or suffer an emotional and mental breakdown.

Then there are those who are simply addicted to working in extreme situations. There is an adrenaline rush, a chemical hit given to them by their own bodies when they have impacted the life of another in a positive way. This is a fortunate side effect otherwise they would have left the important work they do a long time ago.

I have known and worked with all of these people. While there are many articles and books about caring for caregivers, and many organisations write policies and documents for their staff on 'looking after yourself,' I hope this book will strengthen and assist you to discover the unique gifts that you have as a trauma worker and how to make sure you thrive both in your work and in your life.

Challenges for trauma workers

While developing this book I asked experienced trauma workers who are also trauma survivors themselves what their main challenges are. Their responses covered a broad range of personal, professional, interpersonal, and workplace issues. I have grouped these into the following themes as a way of summarising this wealth of information:

Personal

- Re-traumatisation
- Development of and/or increase in personal mental health issues
- Painful exposure to trauma on an ongoing basis
- Feeling as though the world is not a safe place anymore for themselves or for loved ones
- Profound loneliness — you often cannot share your work with others
- Deep emotional fatigue/drain — just becoming more and more tired
- The ongoing reliving of their own trauma and having to manage their own trauma in a conscious way so that it does not affect their clients
- Maintaining a personal self-care routine and ensuring their own self-esteem is not affected
- Being triggered by hearing client stories

Professional

- Counter-transference towards their clients; that is, seeing similarities that can impact upon their professionalism
- Not being able to separate their story from their client's story and potentially projecting their own traumatic experiences onto others
- Believing that what worked for them will work for others without recognising that the client is a different person with different needs and skills
- Their competence - questioning whether they are there for their competence and skills or because they have faced the same experience

- Respecting that other people's experiences of trauma is different to their own

Interpersonal

- Hearing the clients' stories
- Difficulty connecting with other people
- Questioning their own personal life

Workplace

- Leads to exiting from the field due to the difficulty in maintaining a career in trauma work

The greatest challenges

When asked what the greatest challenges are for trauma workers who are trauma survivors themselves, respondents commented:

- Separating their story from others; that is, being entwined with their clients' experiences
- Transference as it impacts their professionalism, their boundaries, vicarious trauma and themselves
- Re-traumatisation as it exacerbates them leaving the field and can lead to development of mental health issues
- The continuous exposure to trauma as it can undermine their sense of the world being a safe place
- Connectedness, as this is at the basis of being able to connect to others/self and possibly a spiritual life
- The profound loneliness of trauma and one's vulnerability in facing it
- The deep emotional impact creating fatigue in all areas of one's life

I will explore these themes further throughout this book.

Issues for trauma workers in their workplaces

Much of my consulting, training and supervision is with early career social workers, psychologists, and counsellors working in the trauma field. They are bright, young, skilled practitioners who work in mainstream government services or in non-government organisations as well as in faith-based organisations.

Their insights about their work are informed by their own life experiences as well as their up-to-date education which, for social workers at least, combines strong human rights and social justice perspectives mixed with policy, practice, and research perspectives. These practitioners are often a welcome addition to organisations taking on newly funded areas of work such as refugees, asylum-seekers, homelessness, domestic violence, sexual assault, and institutional abuses (to name a few). However there are several key challenges I see occurring for these early career practitioners:

- They can speak up about issues in the organisation and this is not always well received by their managers and peers.
- Despite their more recent (and at times better) education than some of their peers and managers, they can be dismissed because they are perceived as 'new' or 'just too young.'
- Although they are enthusiastic about what they do, they are unclear about the next steps to take in their career.
- They have ideas and projects they want to pursue and find it difficult to negotiate the time in their workplaces to do projects to build their own credibility as well as that of their organisations.
- They switch roles in their organisations into new work areas to obtain experience and thus feel they do not become skilled in anything specific.
- They raise ethical matters not only in their own organisations but also in their stakeholder organisations but often see these issues being brushed under the carpet.
- They work long hours sometimes with long commutes and receive little recognition.

Team conflicts and achieving a work/life balance are ongoing challenges. They can frequently feel disrespected, they manage in traumatising work settings with high client and organisation demands while trying to progress in their career. They feel undervalued in their organisations, begin to lose confidence and their work life becomes overwhelming. Add to this mix any personal trauma and it is easy to see how the intersection of the above challenges along with the effects of working with trauma survivors can be a perfect storm for trauma workers.

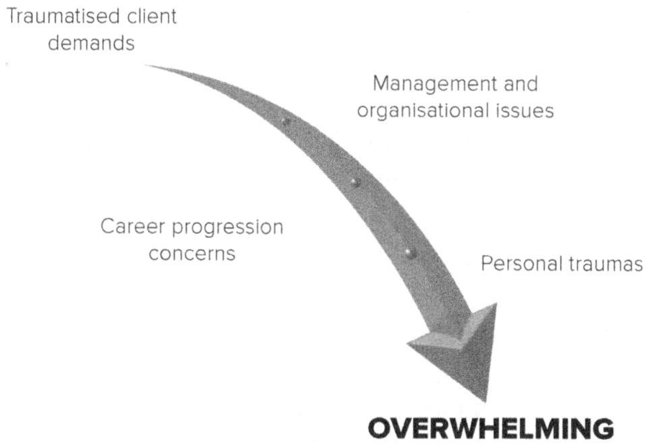

As Peter Levine says in his book 'Healing Trauma' (2008)

> *...trauma is about loss of connection – to ourselves, to our bodies, to our families, to others, and to the world around us. This loss of connection is often hard to recognise, because it doesn't happen all at once. It can happen slowly, over time, and we adapt to these subtle changes sometimes without even noticing them....we may simply sense that we do not feel quite right without ever becoming fully aware of what is taking place; that is, the gradual undermining of our self-esteem, self-confidence, feelings of well-being, and connection to life. (page 9)*

KEY QUESTIONS TO ASK YOURSELF:

Why have I entered trauma work?

What do I wish I could say to people in my work place?

What have I learned from my own life experiences that give me a unique perspective?

What do I love about what I do at work?

What are my key challenges in this workplace?

If I could have two hours a week at work to work on a project for my client group, what would that project be?

What steps could I take to begin to free up two hours a week to work on this project?

Chapter 2

The trauma-filled life

While sorting out some books in my house one day I came across a large, crushed envelope. All that was written on the front of the envelope were two words – 'Letters, Canada.' On opening them I found a copy of two letters my late father had sent to his cousins who were living in Canada.

My father had been contacted by one of his cousins (whom he had never met) and was answering questions posed about his family history. Specifically what my father knew about the life his uncle had in Scotland before he moved to Canada. My father had kept copies of his replies full of rich family stories.

One letter detailed his uncle's experience in Singapore when he was captured and became a Prisoner of War. It detailed some of the torture his uncle had experienced and it was clear from the tone of the letter that my father was deeply moved and very sad. It occurred to me that ordinary families have experienced generations of trauma.

My father wrote about his own grief and sense of loss and disconnection from his family exacerbated by his migration to Australia. Neither of my parents really overcame their sense of loss of family after they migrated to Australia.

While liking the choice they made, it was always bittersweet, especially for my mother who discovered the day she arrived in Australia in April, 1960, that her father had died the week after she left Scotland. Her father had told her it would kill him if she left Scotland with my sister and me. My mother never resolved this grief.

A former colleague of mine, June Huntington, wrote about 'migration as bereavement'. The profound loss people feel living in places where no-one knew them 'back then' and the need to refine and rediscover one's self in a new place finding a sense of 'as-if-ness'. When I worked with June in the early 1980s I remember her telling me that horse riding in Australia gave her a feeling of 'as-if-ness' similar to how she felt when walking on a cold day in England.

When families have been impacted by war as generations have with grandparents, parents, uncles, aunts, sisters and brothers having lived through and witnessed horrors and persecutions, it is the rare person whose life has never been impacted by trauma. Some of the traumas in my family include:

- Wartime deaths
- Wartime imprisonment and torture
- Deaths of babies
- Deaths of children through illness
- Miscarriages
- Divorces
- Sexual assault and abuse
- Family violence
- Assault of a child
- Heart attacks
- Strokes
- Disappearance of a child lasting more than a decade
- Male to female gender reassignment

Despite more recent developments in Australia around trauma and the implementation of trauma-informed care, I find many trauma workers speak in hushed tones about their own personal trauma. Some of this is due to personal privacy concerns in their workplaces where they have to consider career development. When I tell people about my work supporting trauma workers they frequently lean toward me and whisper, 'I am a trauma survivor'.

The whisper is soft and low and the topic changes quickly. What creates this sense of shame and embarrassment? I recently spoke with a counsellor from an organisation where monthly supervision is held for small groups of staff. She commented, 'I have gone to this meeting monthly since I arrived here. We talk about cases which is good. Not once have I heard any of us talk about the impact of a client on us. We don't do that here. The supervisor just listens and doesn't give us any opinion. I suppose it is good that we get supervision. But there is more that we could do.' This clearly indicates a lack of support and understanding for the trauma workers themselves.

I adapted one of the tools I sometimes use with trauma workers from international psychologist and psychodramatist, Dr Kate Hudgins. Kate lives in the USA and is a psychodrama trainer and facilitator. I met her when she visited Australia in the late 1990s and we immediately connected and made plans to work together. Kate had been a psychodramatist for many years and developed a way of using psychodrama with trauma survivors that was less re-traumatising than standard psychodrama approaches. She called her model the 'Therapeutic Spiral.' She outlines in her book 'Experiential Treatment of PTSD' (2002) the importance of strength building for anyone who has experienced trauma. Kate believes that people need to be able to find strength qualities at different levels, and be able to concretise these before they even begin to talk about their traumatic story. These levels are: the personal; the interpersonal; and the transpersonal. I proposed to Kate that a cultural level needs to be added and have found this to be useful for people in multicultural countries like Australia. It is an exercise that can be used individually and in groups, in clinical work, and in supervision sessions.

Let me share a story of how I use this working with trauma workers:

Bella (not her real name) contacted me as she felt she was 'not coping.' She had a client, Delia, who had been severely brutalised throughout her life and Bella was providing her with support about twice a week. Bella had become worried because, on the one hand she knew she was working effectively with Delia and seemed to understand her, but on the other hand Bella was thinking more and more about her own traumatic experiences earlier in her life. She was not sleeping well, not exercising, had put on a lot of weight, had relationship problems at home, and was becoming increasingly depressed. 'I used to be able to keep work and home separate but I don't seem to be able to anymore.'

Initially Bella could not describe any of her own strengths. As we explored further, Bella described herself as caring and associated the colour purple with her style of caring.

She described her cultural strength as laughter. 'Where I grew up you just laughed and got through it. There was no use moaning.' She described herself as non-religious and eventually identified her transpersonal strength as 'nature'. With her marriage about to end she struggled to identify an interpersonal strength and eventually talked about the relationship she had with her dog and the trust that was between them. I talked with Bella about ways she could use each of these elements when making the transition from working with Delia to leaving work and getting back to herself and her own home and family at the end of the day. Bella identified that she could wear something purple, watch more comedy in the evenings after work, and take her dog walking more.

A few days later Bella contacted me and let me know the strategies were helping her at work and at home. Defining her strengths reconnected her to herself, assisted her to support Delia, helped her to maintain better boundaries between Delia and herself, and between her work and home lives.

KEY QUESTIONS TO ASK YOURSELF:

Think of a personal strength — what word, sound, colour, object do you associate with this strength?

Think of an interpersonal strength — what word, sound, colour, object do you associate with this strength?

Think of a cultural strength — what word, sound, colour, object do you associate with this strength?

Note: You may wish to define your cultural strength as related to the culture of your family, the place you grew up, or you may identify more than one strength if you lived in different countries or your parents and family members had different cultural backgrounds.

Think of a transpersonal strength — what word, sound, colour, object do you associate with this strength? This can be challenging for some people to articulate. Some people may link it to their religious or spiritual traditions while others may be unclear about what 'transpersonal' is. I often refine it by asking, 'what is the strength or quality beyond all others that keeps you alive, that gives you your will to live?'

Chapter 3

What is trauma?

According to the Oxford English Dictionary the word 'trauma' is derived from the Greek meaning 'wound.' It can refer to a deeply disturbing experience, an emotional shock after a stressful event that can lead to long term consequences, or a physical injury. In each case it is something that happens to someone from an outside event or experience and the event can be re-lived in the future which further adds to the trauma. Each individual's response to trauma can be as unique as each person. However we do know that over time trauma can impact us more and more even many years after the original events.

People who come forward and speak of horrific child abuse often speak of how the memories have never left them. Some say they became stronger for their experiences; others speak of being destroyed and having 'shattered lives.' Eric was a man in his 80s who had suffered physical, emotional and sexual abuse as a child while in an orphanage after the death of his mother. He wept as he recounted, 'I have had 70 jobs in my life. I was an A-grade student then all **that** [referring to the abuses] happened at school and I never achieved. All my life I thought it was something deficient in me. I didn't trust people. I thought it was me.'

Different types of trauma

When considering the types of trauma that survivors experience it is clear that there is a huge range of traumatic experiences both workers and survivors may share in their lives.

- **Single event traumatic experiences** — this often relates to something unplanned, unexpected, and overwhelming. An accident, an individual experience of abuse or assault, a disaster, the sudden death of someone close to you, or witnessing an act of violence against another person.
- **Complex traumatic experiences** — this refers to situations where the abuse or trauma is ongoing or is repeated frequently. Situations can include living through a war, or experiencing on-going domestic violence/sexual abuse over many years.
- **Developmental traumatic experiences** — this refers to traumatic experiences people may have experienced from a very young age that is repeated during childhood or adolescence. Repeated instances of physical abuse, sexual abuse, neglect, abandonment, deaths in the family along with experiences where caregivers for the child or young person are neglectful may lead to the child experiencing interruptions in the care they receive during their formative years. This may affect the person's ability to form healthy caring attachments with others, potentially harming relationships later in life. There are, of course, many people who do find a way to create a different life for their own children.
- **Intergenerational traumatic experiences** — some people and their families have been exposed to trauma across several generations. The family system has been built around coping with the effects of trauma in other people in the family as well as current traumas. Examples may be families who have lived through war in one or more generations and are trying to rebuild their lives after the losses of family members, and/or loss of country (see also historical trauma). Many people develop unique personal responses to surviving trauma and may pass on their coping mechanisms to other family members even when the traumatic events no longer exist.
- **Historical traumatic experiences** — have frequently happened to large groups of people across land and time. Examples are people who have lived through human trafficking, slavery, extensive wartime experiences and genocide.

We would be hard pressed to find a trauma worker who has never been exposed to some of the traumas summarised above. Simply living our lives means we will be exposed to significant life events.

Why should we care about trauma?

Many years ago people 'toughed it out' or would say to themselves, 'other people experience much worse situations.' While this helped people build on their strengths and ways they could make a better life for themselves and their families, we now know that trauma affects people's physical, psychological emotional, social, and, at times, spiritual wellbeing. People often underestimate the effects of the event and it may not be until later in life they begin to consider (or understand) the impact of the trauma experiences they have lived through. While a response to trauma may be quite individual and unique, the table in the next section gives some of the common reactions people who are trauma survivors may experience.

What parts of me get impacted?

The largest study in the world into the adverse effects of exposure to trauma in childhood was conducted in the USA with over 18,000 participants. This study concluded that where people had high numbers of incidences in their childhood of what is called 'adverse traumatic events' there were significant impacts on their future health and wellbeing.

A scoring system was developed for those who completed the survey and it was concluded that the greater exposure children had to the stresses associated with traumatic events the following health problems could result:

- Alcoholism and alcohol abuse
- Chronic Obstructive Pulmonary Disease (COPD)
- Depression
- Foetal death
- Poor health-related quality of life
- Illicit drug use
- Ischemic Heart Disease (IHD)
- Liver disease
- Risk for intimate partner violence

- Multiple sexual partners
- Sexually Transmitted Diseases (STDs)
- Smoking
- Suicide attempts
- Unintended pregnancies
- Early initiation of smoking
- Early initiation of sexual activity
- Adolescent pregnancy

Rarely do we hear medical practitioners linking these physical health issues to earlier experiences of trauma. We are naïve if we expect trauma workers not to have experienced some adverse childhood and adulthood events also.

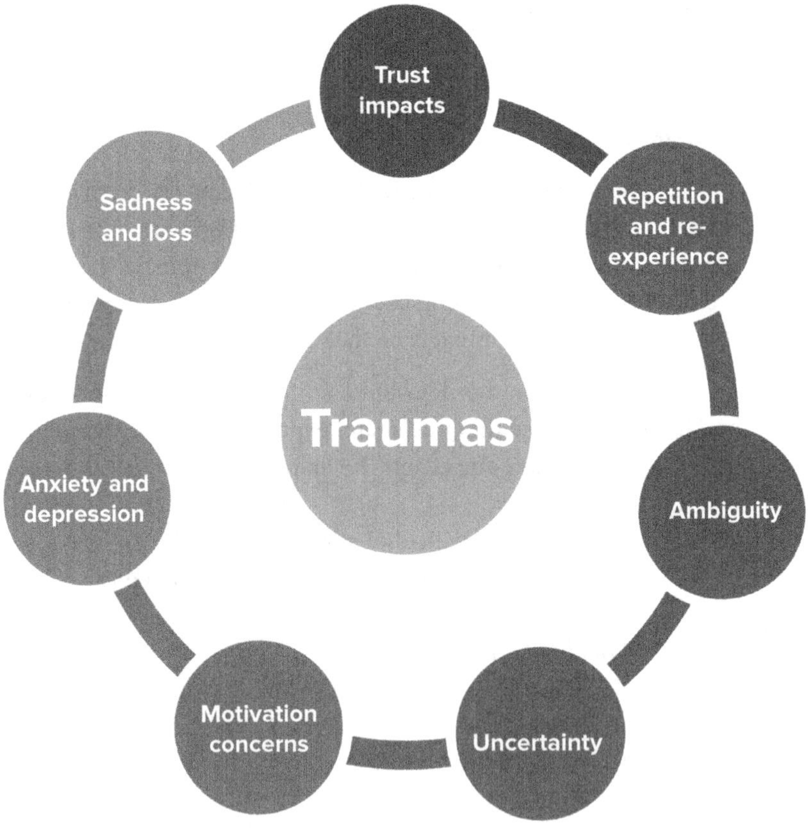

T rauma impacts us physically, emotionally, mentally, and psychologically.

R epetition and re-experiencing can occur immediately, as well as many years after a traumatic experience.

A mbiguity occurs when we feel as though we are living in two worlds. It also occurs when we have a sense that those who care about us are physically present and psychologically absent (such as family members with depression), or physically absent and psychologically present (such as a missing family member). Finding meaning, tempering mastery, reconstructing identities, and discovering hope are all necessary. *(Boss, 2006)*

U ncertainty occurs during and after traumas. We may not know the immediate or long-term impacts on our lives.

M otivational concerns — living with the effects of traumas can make us exhausted and unclear about how to respond to or overcome the traumatic event.

A nxiety and depression can occur after a trauma and may need clinical management by a doctor, social worker, psychologist, counsellor or psychiatrist. Complementary medicine practitioners may also assist.

S adness and loss may result depending on the trauma as well as simply due to the trauma. Feeling sad for ourselves and what we have lost can be a part of the process of managing the trauma and can sometimes have a surprising consequence.

IMPACT OF TRAUMA

BODY SYSTEM	REACTION
Physical	Alcoholism Asthma Auto-immune issues Brain development changes Chronic fatigue Gastro-intestinal problems Headaches Immune system issues Listlessness Musculoskeletal problems Ongoing chronic pain Palpitations in the heart
Psychological	Anxiety Flashbacks Hyperarousal Intrusive thoughts Memory loss Nightmares Shock
Emotional	Difficulties controlling emotions Helplessness Numbness Powerlessness Shame Terror
Social	Feeling disconnected from others Hypervigilance with self and others
Spiritual	Loss of faith in life

KEY QUESTIONS TO ASK YOURSELF:

What physical issues do I experience on a regular basis?

What psychological issues are increasing for me?

What emotional issues am I having in my work and my life?

What changes have occurred in my social and personal relationships since working in trauma work?

How do I keep my own spirit alive among the traumatic experiences to which I bear witness either directly or indirectly?

Chapter 4

How does trauma get assessed?

This section focuses on some of the tools used to assess trauma. Many people are familiar with the tool developed by Drs Thomas Holmes and Richard Rahe to help people to identify their potential stress quotient.

They developed this tool after interviewing over 7000 people and devising numerical rankings for the events that people perceived to be stressful. By completing the questionnaire about the number of stressful events that you have experienced in the last 12 months, it is possible to identify whether you are likely to need further assistance and support.

When people are living through several life changes at once, they often forget that even positive events can carry a stress loading. The following has been adapted from their survey. You can develop your score through placing the 'Stress quotient event value' from the third column into the 'Your score' column if you have experienced this event in the last 12 months.

LIFE EVENT	Happened to you in the last 12 months	Stress quotient event value	SCORE
Death of a spouse	No Yes	100	
Divorce	No Yes	73	
Marital Separation	No Yes	65	
Detention in jail or an institution	No Yes	63	
Death of close family member	No Yes	63	
Major personal injury or illness	No Yes	53	

LIFE EVENT	Happened to you in the last 12 months		Stress quotient event value	SCORE
Marriage	No	Yes	50	
Being fired at work	No	Yes	47	
Marital reconciliation	No	Yes	45	
Retirement from work	No	Yes	45	
Major change in health or behaviour of a family member	No	Yes	44	
Pregnancy	No	Yes	40	
Sexual difficulty	No	Yes	40	
Gaining a new family member through birth, adoption or remarriage	No	Yes	39	
Major business readjustment	No	Yes	39	
Major change in financial state	No	Yes	38	
Death of a close friend	No	Yes	37	
Change to a different line of work	No	Yes	36	
Major increase in the number of arguments with a spouse	No	Yes	35	
Taking on a mortgage	No	Yes	31	
Foreclosure on a mortgage or loan	No	Yes	30	
Major change in work responsibilities e.g. promotion, demotion or transfer	No	Yes	29	
Son or daughter leaving home	No	Yes	29	
Trouble with in–laws	No	Yes	29	
Outstanding personal achievement	No	Yes	28	
Spouse beginning or ending their work outside the home	No	Yes	26	
Going back to school/university	No	Yes	26	
Major change in living conditions i.e. renovating or significant deterioration in your home	No	Yes	25	
Revision of personal daily lifestyle habits	No	Yes	24	
Problems with superiors at work	No	Yes	23	
Major changes in working hours or conditions	No	Yes	20	

LIFE EVENT	Happened to you in the last 12 months		Stress quotient event value	SCORE
Changing where you live	No	Yes	20	
Major change in type or amount of recreation	No	Yes	19	
Major change in regular religious activity	No	Yes	19	
Major change in social activities	No	Yes	18	
Purchase of a car or other major expenditure	No	Yes	17	
Major change in sleeping habits	No	Yes	16	
Major change in number of family get-togethers	No	Yes	15	
Major change in eating habits	No	Yes	15	
Having a vacation	No	Yes	13	
Christmas or holiday observances	No	Yes	12	
Minor violations of the law e.g. traffic tickets	No	Yes	11	
TOTAL SCORE				

Results:

Your total score indicates the possible risks of having a physical illness in the next 12 months:

100–199 — mild risk
200–299 — moderate risk
300 or more — strong risk

There are a number of other tools available which can assist trauma workers who are trauma survivors themselves to identify some of the traumas that they have experienced and what may be currently impacting upon them now. In my work, it is common to see trauma workers with increased alcohol consumption, multiple relationship breakdowns, and issues with family/children/workplace relationships. Often these are put down to the stresses of work or just life in general. Being more self-reflective and bringing an awareness to some of the experiences that trauma workers have had in their own past may assist in identifying strategies to reduce their impact in their present and future lives.

Brief Trauma Questionnaire (BTQ)

This questionnaire was developed from a Brief Trauma Interview schedule. It is helpful in assisting people to assess whether they meet the trauma exposure criteria for Post-Traumatic Stress Disorder in earlier versions of the Diagnostic and Statistical Manual of the American Psychiatric Association. It helps to assess threats to life, or serious injury, in relation to exposure to traumatic events.

It asks questions about extraordinarily stressful or disturbing events which most people would react to. If the participant indicates that they have experienced an event then they are also asked about the impact on their life in terms of serious injuries or potential fatalities.

HAS THIS EVER HAPPENED TO YOU?

Event	Response	Threat to life/fear of serious injury	Actual serious injury
1 Have you ever served in a war zone, or have you ever served in a non-combat job that exposed you to war-related casualties (for example, as a medic or graves registration duty)?	No Yes	No Yes	No Yes
2 Have you been in a serious car accident, or a serious accident at work or somewhere else?	No Yes	No Yes	No Yes
3 Have you ever been in a major natural or technological disaster, such as a fire, tornado, hurricane, flood, earthquake, or chemical spill?	No Yes	No Yes	No Yes
4 Have you ever had a life-threatening illness such as cancer, a heart attack, leukaemia, AIDS, Multiple Sclerosis etc?	No Yes	No Yes	No Yes
5 Before age 18, were you physically punished or beaten by a parent, caretaker, or teacher so that: you were very frightened or you thought you would be injured or you received bruises, cuts, welts, lumps or other injuries?	No Yes	No Yes	No Yes
6 (NOT including any punishments or beatings you already reported in question 5) **Have you ever been attacked, beaten, or mugged by anyone, including friends, family members, or strangers?**	No Yes	No Yes	No Yes

Event	Response	Threat to life/fear of serious injury	Actual serious injury
7 Has anyone ever made or pressured you into having some type of unwanted sexual contact? Note: Sexual contact here means any contact between someone else and your private body areas or between you and someone else's private body parts	No Yes	No Yes	No Yes
8 Have you ever been in any other situation in which you were seriously injured, or have you been in any other situation in which you feared you might be seriously injured or killed?	No Yes	No Yes	No Yes
9 Has a close family member or friend died violently, for example, in a serious car crash, mugging or attack?	No Yes	No Yes	No Yes
10 Have you ever witnessed a situation in which someone was seriously injured or killed, or have you ever witnessed a situation in which you feared someone would be seriously injured or killed? Note: Do not answer 'yes' for any event you have already reported in questions 1–9	No Yes	No Yes	No Yes

Impact of Events Scale (IES)

This scale was developed by Mardi Horowitz, Nancy Wilner and William Alvarez in 1979. It assists in assessing the impact of traumatic events by checking in on the distress that people are experiencing as a result of the event. After listing the current date, the date of the traumatic event and writing a brief description of the event, provide a response to the following comments based on your experience over the last seven days:

In the last 7 days:	Not At All	Rarely	Sometimes	Often
I have thought about it when I didn't mean to	0	1	3	5
I avoided letting myself get upset when I thought about it or was reminded about it	0	1	3	5
I tried to remove it from my memory	0	1	3	5
I had trouble falling asleep or staying asleep because of pictures/ thoughts about it	0	1	3	5

In the last 7 days:	Not At All	Rarely	Sometimes	Often
I had waves of strong feelings about it	0	1	3	5
I had dreams about it	0	1	3	5
I stayed away from reminders of it	0	1	3	5
I felt as if it hadn't happened or was unreal	0	1	3	5
I tried not to talk about it	0	1	3	5
Images of it popped into my mind	0	1	3	5
I had other things that kept making me think about it	0	1	3	5
I was aware that I still had a lot of feelings about it, but I didn't deal with them	0	1	3	5
I tried not to think about it	0	1	3	5
I had reminders that brought back feelings about it	0	1	3	5
My feelings about it were kind of numb	0	1	3	5
Scores – add up each column	0	+	+	+
TOTAL STRESS SCORE add results of each column				

Score of 0–8 means there is currently no meaningful impact of the event

Score of 19–25 means there is some impact and you may be affected

Score of 26–43 means you have been greatly affected by the event

Score of 44–75 means you are likely to have severe impact due to the event

Post-Traumatic Stress Disorder (PTSD) is a specific diagnosis with scores of 27 on this scale indicating you might have some symptoms of PTSD. Scores 35–75 indicate that you are likely to meet the criteria for PTSD.

Trauma and Beliefs Scale

This scale, developed by Drs Laurie Anne Perlman and I. Lisa McCann, is used in some organisations to assist trauma workers to monitor changes that may develop in their thinking due to being exposed to trauma. It monitors the following self-trust/other trust; self-esteem/other esteem; self-safety/other safety; and self-intimacy/other intimacy. Some organisations use this scale with trauma workers to facilitate monitoring of vicarious trauma levels. However, the original scale was developed for psychotherapeutic work with clients.

Professional Quality of Life Scale (PROQOL)

This scale, developed by Dr Beth Hudnall Stamm, is used by trauma workers to monitor compassion, satisfaction, burnout, and compassion fatigue. Consider the following statements and think about how frequently you have experienced these in the last 30 days:

Statement	1 Never	2 Rarely	3 Sometimes	4 Often	5 Very Often
1. I am happy					
2. I am preoccupied with more than one person that I help					
3. I get satisfaction from being able to help people					
4. I feel connected to others					
5. I jump or am startled by unexpected sounds					
6. I feel invigorated after working with those I help					
7. I find it difficult to separate my personal life from my life as a helper					
8. I am not as productive at work because I am losing sleep over traumatic experiences of people I help					
9. I think that I might have been affected by the traumatic stress of those I help					
10. I feel trapped by my job as a helper					

Statement	1 Never	2 Rarely	3 Sometimes	4 Often	5 Very Often
11. Because of my helping, I have felt 'on edge' about various things					
12. I like my work as a helper					
13. I feel depressed because of the traumatic experiences of the people I help					
14. I feel as though I am experiencing the trauma of someone I have helped					
15. I have beliefs that sustain me					
16. I am pleased with how I am able to keep up with helping techniques and protocols					
17. I am the person that I always wanted to be					
18. My work makes me feel satisfied					
19. I feel worn out because of my work as a helper					
20. I have happy thoughts and feelings about those I help and how I could help them					
21. I feel overwhelmed because my case workload seems endless					
22. I believe I can make a difference through my work					
23. I avoid certain activities or situations because they remind me of the frightening experiences of the people I help					
24. I am proud of what I can do to help					
25. As a result of my helping, I have intrusive, frightening thoughts					
26. I feel 'bogged down' by the system					

Statement	1 Never	2 Rarely	3 Sometimes	4 Often	5 Very Often
27. I have thoughts that I am a 'success' as a helper					
28. I can't recall important parts of my work with trauma victims					
29. I am a very caring person					
30. I am happy I chose the work I am doing					
TOTAL SCORE					

What the scores mean...

COMPASSION SATISFACTION SCALE

Add the responses to questions 3, 6, 12, 16, 18, 20, 22, 24, 27, 30. The total means:

Sum of COMPASSION SATISFACTION questions	Score Equals	Compassion Satisfaction Level
22 or Less	43 or Less	Low
Between 23-41	Around 50	Average
42 or More	57 or More	High

BURNOUT SCALE

Reverse the scoring for questions 1, 4, 15, 17, 29 then add in the scores for questions 8, 10, 19, 21, and 26. The total means:

Sum of BURNOUT questions	Score Equals	Burnout Level
22 or Less	43 or Less	Low
Between 23-41	Around 50	Average
42 or More	57 or More	High

SECONDARY TRAUMATIC STRESS SCALE

The total for questions 2, 5, 7, 9, 11, 13, 14, 23, 25, 28 means:

Sum of SECONDARY TRAUMA questions	Score Equals	Secondary Traumatic Stress Levels
22 or Less	43 or Less	Low
Between 23-41	Around 50	Average
42 or More	57 or More	High

KEY QUESTIONS TO ASK YOURSELF:

What tool did you find most useful?

How can you build in a reminder to test yourself at least twice a year?

What changes can you make to your daily work/life program to reduce impacts of trauma on yourself?

Chapter 5

Is it mind over body or body over mind?

In her book 'Molecules of Emotion' scientist Candace Pert outlined her work in developing the field of psycho-neuro-immunology. Simply put, this is how mechanisms in our body translate how we think into chemical changes in our bodies that subsequently affect our immune system.

Bessel van der Kolk is known worldwide in the trauma field for his work in identifying the effects of the brain affected by trauma. Research into trauma and its effects is still a burgeoning field and whilst knowing the effects on the brain and body is important and useful, it still leaves people wondering what it means for them.

Many trauma workers who are also trauma survivors had no control over what happened to them in their lives (particularly as children) and the focus on the problems that they are likely to have as a result can further undermine their confidence and self-esteem.

I remember sitting at university listening to lectures providing the data about the type of family I came from and noting how few people ever succeeded. At the time I felt that I could not 'own up' to what was happening in my own family then. I needed to work harder to show competence and 'normality'. I notice as I teach at university now in social work and medicine that students are often more prepared to be open about their experiences.

They seek out and use some of the support now available at universities and tertiary education programs such as learning centres, and equity and disability services.

Many trauma workers who are also trauma survivors do take a mind over body attitude to their experiences. 'I just got on with it,' I hear people say, or 'if I wasn't prepared to help myself then who else would?' They work hard, often to the detriment of their own health, family and personal relationships.

I remember how one morning, after experiencing 18 months of court cases following the sexual assault of one of my daughters by a stranger, combined with a further 18 months of legal matters to restore access to her after she was taken by my ex-husband at 14 years of age, I woke up just knowing I could not face going to work.

I called in sick. Then I got dressed, went outside and began to walk. I walked and walked and walked and walked. Gazing in shop windows, strolling through shops, I kept on walking. The feeling of my feet touching the footpath seemed to keep me alive in some way. I reflected on a client with schizophrenia whom I had treated many years earlier who described how 'he just had to walk.' I experienced that same feeling that day. My body needed to keep on going no matter what. Eight hours later I returned home.

The next day I went to see my GP who reminded me I was experiencing delayed grief after all that had happened in the court cases. Another client I had described how she experienced uncontrollable shaking after a series of particularly traumatic events over many years. 'It was like my body just had to shake everything out,' she said. Peter Levine describes this as a common response to overwhelming trauma.

Recent developments in brain imaging through the use of Magnetic Resonance Imaging techniques (MRIs) enable us to identify areas of the brain and body that are affected by traumatic events. This demonstrates that trauma responses occur in the body as well as in the mind and affects the ways in which we change and relate to others and often to ourselves.

One day, Australian poet Jennifer Maiden was visiting my house with her husband and daughter. As I was preparing for dinner, my four year old daughter Tessa leaned on the table on her elbows, swinging her feet up off the floor, and called out, 'Look Jenny, I am standing on no floor.'

We all laughed at the time and Jenny then used those words in the following poem. It details some of the ways that people experience and try to make sense of trauma.

Some of the women noted in this poem had experienced abuse as children as well as in adult relationships and the Aboriginal poet Dennis McDermott once told me it was the best poem he had read addressing these issues.

Look, I'm Standing on No-Floor

said Margaret Cunningham's four-
year-old daughter Tessa, her fingers
clenched whitely on the table-edge, her feet
luxuriously in air. Margaret is still Director
of STARRTS, the N.S.W. Service for Torture
and Trauma Rehab., and I am still their
sort of Writer-on-Call. Together
we wrote a chapter about a child
called Layla who comes from no-country
in particular, a fact which has already —
together with the letterhead Torture and Trauma —
put off at least one publisher. Layla
has witnessed torture and many other
forms of not-belonging. Margaret and I often
have also stood on no-floor, child or woman.

After Tessa
said that, I joked about the shoes
I'd worn the day before: open high-heels
very black and very tall, and very
precarious: "I was standing on no-floor
a lot yesterday", but it was
worth it because I only paid nine
dollars for the sandals and felt as sexy
as something airy from another world.
But the torture:
Margaret joked about a phone call
to the T.&T. Unit from the cloistered A.B.C.,
asking to interview clients who'd really
enjoyed their torture, were into S-M. I
observed this was a travesty of my theory

that people after trauma need a hierarchy
but both idealize and demonize it, and that
recognition of S–M in their sexuality
might clarify the process for them:
hell,
when you're standing on no–floor, you skate
or fall or just stay–put, appreciate
the elevation. We also spoke of Arthur
Stieglitz photographing Georgia O'Keeffe
as hundreds of nudes, and how women at one
of Margaret's workshops had gone out to pay
a photographer to give them back their bodies.
One works better in all areas, I think, with
a confidence in one's geography,
and if
there's a vaginal velvet emptiness at centre
studded with that vaginal
diamond mine of nerves,
no–floor is not a life–defining problem.
On the wall
near this table at Margaret's, a Georgia
O'Keeffe lily is as poised as Tessa's joy.

KEY QUESTIONS TO ASK YOURSELF:

Think about a trauma that you have experienced:

How did your body react at the time?

What were your thoughts?

What beliefs did you develop?

What decisions have you made since that occasion?

How do your body's responses support you?

Chapter 6

What does it mean to thrive?

To 'thrive' means to grow, or develop, to prosper and to flourish. It is derived from a Middle Norse word meaning to grow or increase. Many people do thrive and grow beyond their traumatic experiences and this is a testament to the many trauma survivors who become successful in their chosen career, life, and relationships. A man who had survived child sexual assault said, 'one thing I learned was the way I was never going to be and I have been a good father to my children and grandchildren.'

Writers such as Viktor Frankl speak about the importance of finding meaning in traumatic experiences. He was interned as a Prisoner of War during World War Two and in his book 'Man's Search for Meaning' he says, 'life is never made unbearable by circumstances, but only by lack of meaning and purpose.' The world also marvels at men like Nelson Mandela and the Dalai Lama, both of whom have suffered terribly yet inspire generations with their messages of peace, hope, compassion, love and forgiveness towards those who harm them. Trauma workers have many such heroes and heroines including those mentioned above. From those who responded to the survey, heroes included the following:

- Family members;
- People in specific professions, such as nurses, police officers, or public servants who stood up and spoke out against injustices;
- Faculty members, such as school teachers or school principals;

- People related to their workplace and professional support, such as an executive officer where they work, their clients, or a professional mentor; and
- People in public leadership positions, such as General Peter Cosgrove (current Governor-General of Australia).

Then there were also specific individuals included in the list from a wide range of fields who inspire trauma workers, including:

Maya Angelou - American author and social commentator. Below is one of her most famous poems:

Still I rise

You may write me down in history

With your bitter, twisted lies,
You may trod me in the very dirt
But still, like dust, I'll rise.

Does my sassiness upset you?
Why are you beset with gloom?
'Cause I walk like I've got oil wells
Pumping in my living room.

Just like moons and like suns,
With the certainty of tides,
Just like hopes springing high,
Still I'll rise.

Did you want to see me broken?
Bowed head and lowered eyes?
Shoulders falling down like teardrops.
Weakened by my soulful cries.

Does my haughtiness offend you?
Don't you take it awful hard
'Cause I laugh like I've got gold mines
Diggin' in my own back yard.

You may shoot me with your words,
You may cut me with your eyes,
You may kill me with your hatefulness,
But still, like air, I'll rise.

Does my sexiness upset you?
Does it come as a surprise
That I dance like I've got diamonds
At the meeting of my thighs?

Out of the huts of history's shame
I rise
Up from a past that's rooted in pain
I rise
I'm a black ocean, leaping and wide,
Welling and swelling I bear in the tide.
Leaving behind nights of terror and fear
I rise
Into a daybreak that's wondrously clear
I rise
Bringing the gifts that my ancestors gave,
I am the dream and the hope of the slave.
I rise
I rise
I rise.

Elie Weisel – a holocaust survivor and Nobel Peace Prize winner who spoke out for peace and I believe that our personal responsibility to speak up is mirrored in his quote:

There may be times when we are powerless to prevent injustice,
but there must never be a time when we fail to protest.

Virginia Satir – social worker who developed a model of family therapy based on the importance of love and helping people to become their authentic self. Below is her famous poem:

I am me – A Declaration of Self-Esteem

In all the world there is not one exactly like me.

Everything that comes out of me is authentically mine because
I choose it

I own everything about me, my body, my feelings, my mouth, my voice, all my actions whether they be to others or to myself

I own my fantasies, my dreams, my hopes, my fears

I own all of my triumphs and successes, all of my failures and mistakes

because I own all of me. I become intimately acquainted with me...by so doing, I can love me and be friendly with me in all my parts

I know there are aspects about myself that puzzle me and other aspects I do not know...but as long as I am friendly and loving to myself, I can courageously and hopefully look for solutions to the puzzles and for ways to find out more about me...

however I look and sound whatever I say and do, and whatever I think and feel at a given moment in time is authentically me...

if later some parts of how I looked, sounded, thought and felt turned out to be unfitting, I can discard that which is unfitting and keep the rest and invest something new for that which I discard...I can see, hear, feel, think, say and do.

I have the tools to survive, to be close to others, to be productive, and to make sense and order out of the world of people and things outside of me...I own me and therefore I can engineer me...

I am me and **I AM OKAY.**

Hannah Arendt - the 20th century Jewish philosopher who wrote about what was happening in Germany during World War II. She is known for some of her quotes on forgiveness such as, *'Forgiveness is the key to action and freedom'*; her comments on evil, *'The sad truth is that most evil is done by people who never make up their minds to be good or evil'*; and ways we should live, *'Dedicate yourself to the good you deserve and desire for yourself. Give yourself peace of mind. You deserve to be happy. You deserve to delight.'*

Immortal Technique - the Peruvian rapper based in Harlem, New York who retains control over his music and production and uses his music for social commentary, such as his song *'Dance with the Devil'* which encourages young men not to enter a life of crime.

Nick Kristof - the Pulitzer prize winning journalist who writes regular opinion pieces in the New York Times and raised human rights violations in his book *'Half the sky: Turning Oppression into Opportunity for Women Worldwide'* which focusses on the oppression of women and girls in developing countries.

Margaret Atwood - the Canadian poet, novelist and literary critic. She is also an environmental activist and author of the following poem:

Love

This is a word we use to plug
holes with. It's the right size for those warm
blanks in speech, for those red heart-
shaped vacancies on the page that look nothing
like real hearts. Add lace
and you can sell
it. We insert it also in the one empty
space on the printed form
that comes with no instructions. There are whole
magazines with not much in them
but the word love, you can
rub it all over your body and you
can cook with it too. How do we know
it isn't what goes on at the cool
debaucheries of slugs under damp
pieces of cardboard? As for the weed-
seedlings nosing their tough snouts up
among the lettuces, they shout it.
Love! Love! sing the soldiers, raising
their glittering knives in salute.

Then there's the two
of us. This word
is far too short for us, it has only
four letters, too sparse
to fill those deep bare
vacuums between the stars
that press on us with their deafness.
It's not love we don't wish
to fall into, but that fear.
this word is not enough but it will
have to do. It's a single
vowel in this metallic
silence, a mouth that says
O again and again in wonder
and pain, a breath, a finger
grip on a cliffside. You can
hold on or let go.

Sonia Sotomayor - the first Hispanic woman to become a US Supreme Court judge and author of the book *'My Beloved World.'* As she says: *'I do know one thing about me: I don't measure myself by others' expectations or let others define my worth.'* She believes firmly that until *'there is equality of education there is no equality.'*

Joan Baez — the American folk singer, song-writer and activist whose songs inspired non-violent movements. She is quoted as saying, *'Action is the antidote to despair'* and, *'you don't get to choose how you're going to die, or when. You can only decide how you're going to live. Now.'*

Nelson Mandela - the lawyer who became President of South Africa. He was jailed for over 27 years for his stand against apartheid. Author of the book *'Long Road to Freedom'* in which he advocates optimism:

> *Part of being optimistic is keeping one's head pointed toward the sun, one's feet moving forward. There were many dark moments when my faith in humanity was sorely tested, but I would not and could not give myself up to despair. That way lays defeat and death.*

Julia Gillard — the first female prime minister of Australia who made an impassioned plea to the Australian parliament regarding misogyny.

David Bohm - the American born British physicist who contributed to philosophy, physics, and neuropsychology. He said, *'The ability to perceive or think differently is more important than the knowledge gained.'*

Mother Theresa - the founder of a catholic missionary group working in India. She is reputed to have written the following:

> *People are often unreasonable, irrational and self-centred. Forgive them anyway.*
>
> *If you are kind, people may accuse you of selfish, ulterior motives. Be kind anyway.*
>
> *If you are successful, you will win some unfaithful friends and some genuine enemies. Succeed anyway.*
>
> *If you are honest and sincere people may deceive you. Be honest and sincere anyway.*
>
> *What you spend years creating, others could destroy overnight. Create anyway.*
>
> *If you find serenity and happiness, some may be jealous. Be happy anyway.*
>
> *The good you do today will often be forgotten. Do good anyway.*
>
> *Give the best you have, and it will never be enough. Give your best anyway.*
>
> *In the final analysis it is between you and God. It was never between you and them anyway.*

Madonna - the American entertainer who became a cultural icon and noted for taking risks in her style of songs and entertainment. She reminds us, *'No matter who you are, no matter what you did, no matter where you've come from, you can always change, become a better version of yourself.'*

Butet Manurung - the woman who campaigns and develops alternative education programs for people living in remote and isolated jungle areas in Indonesia. (See www.onejustworld.com.au/Speakers/Butet-Manurung)

Aung San Suu Kyi - the pro-democracy leader in Burma who was held under house arrest for nearly 15 years.

When awarded the Nobel Prize for Peace in 1991 she said, *'Often during my days of house arrest it felt as though I were no longer a part of the real world. There was the house which was my world, there was the world of others who also were not free but who were together in prison as a community, and there was the world of the free; each was a different planet pursuing its own separate course in an indifferent universe.'*

Mahatma Gandhi — the father of India's independence movement who developed non-violent protest processes and inspired later civil rights leaders such as Martin Luther King Jnr. He is reputed to have said *'you must be the change you wish to see in the world'* as well as *'happiness is when what you think, what you say, and what you do are in harmony.'* He also reminds us to *'Live as if you were to die tomorrow. Learn as if you were to live forever.'*

Jill Scott — the American actress and singer who grew up in the ghetto with her mother and grandmother. She reminds us that *'every individual has his or her own power, and it's a matter of working, taking time and defining what that power is.'* She also talks about the importance of stories in our lives: *'anytime you share life stories with other people, you know you are acknowledging their humanity and kind of accessing some things about yourself, and other people start to expect things about themselves. It's kind of like a fellowship.'* She also reminds us of some things we can do when we are not feeling on top of things: *'If I feel really ugly or unhappy, sometimes I'll choose bright colors so they'll make me feel good. Yellows, pinks, light blues and orange. I just want to feel good all the time if I can.'*

Barack Obama - the first African-American president of the USA campaigned on the changes we can make saying, *'Change will not come if we wait for some other person or some other time. We are the ones we've been waiting for. We are the change we seek.'* He also reminds us to be determined: *'If you are walking down the right path and you are willing to keep walking, eventually you will make progress.'* He also wants people to have a larger ambition for themselves saying, *'Focusing your life solely on making a buck shows a certain poverty of ambition. It asks too little of yourself. Because it's only when you hitch your wagon to something larger than yourself that you realize your true potential.'*

Tim Duncan - the American basketball player who always plays his hardest and says, *'I'm just going to play whatever game is in front of me.'*

Idris Elba — the British actor and musician whose father was Sierra Leonese and mother Ghanian. He reminds us that *'whether it's music or acting, that creativity all comes from the same source.'*

Lady Ga Ga - the performer and entertainer who takes a stand against bullying and wants her music to make a difference in young people's lives. *'Every bit of me is devoted to love and art. And I aspire to try to be a teacher to my young fans who feel just like I felt when I was younger. I just felt like a freak. I guess what I'm trying to say is I'm trying to liberate them, I want to free them of their fears and make them feel that they can make their own space in the world.'* She encourages us to see the good in people: *'I feel like if you're a really good human being, you can try to find something beautiful in every single person, no matter what.'*

Yoko Ono - the artist, musician and singer who performed with her late husband John Lennon. She said, *'Healing yourself is connected with healing others,'* and as one trauma worker remarked, *'people who are themselves and accept others for themselves' are inspiring.*

KEY QUESTIONS TO ASK YOURSELF:

Who are your heroes?

Who are your heroines?

Whose words inspire you the most?

Make a collage using any materials reflecting the inspiration that you receive from your heroes and heroines and show how it impacts upon you.

Chapter 7

How people end up in trauma work

My own story of how I ended up in trauma work is a journey mixed with doses of planning, unplanned surprises, and intriguing synchronicity. As a social worker it is expected that we deal with people in all kinds of situations. In my early career I worked as the first social worker who had worked in a particular state psychiatric hospital for five years.

I had the opportunity to work with the community psychiatrist Dr Donald Scott-Orr who was insightful and challenging and above all educational. I was a keen and avid learner and would listen to him talk for hours on the days he attended the unit. With the development of community health services in Australia, an opportunity arose to become the first community health social worker on the Central Coast of NSW. This was at a time when a new way of working with communities was evolving in Australia and I found myself working with clients in their homes, advising on social work role for aged care services as well as child and family services, donning a PR role as I spoke to media about the need for accommodation services and a women's health service, establishing a local child care services committee, and training the first community educators for the health education program at the time with my friend and mentor Liesel Relf. After the birth of my son, I approached my local medical service suggesting they employ me part-time as a social worker in their practice, initially to develop 'Preparation for Parenthood' classes in an area with young families who had a long drive through country roads to the nearest major hospital.

Fortunately they liked this idea and my role also developed into working with people where a member of the family decided to die at home. This enhanced my skills in working with the terminally ill and their families in an area and time where palliative care services were non-existent.

On returning to Sydney some years later I took up the opportunity to work in the marriage guidance area increasing my skills in working with couples with sexual problems. I then worked as a community health social worker in Penrith, a growing area with few community resources for counselling, for children who needed play therapy, or for couples who were struggling. I developed 'Preparation for Parenthood' classes that in a short time went from 10 to 60 people per session, and created some specific group programs in collaboration with the health education officer.

With a young family of my own, I moved into a senior social worker role in a larger community health centre with a more extensive range of services across five suburbs, and thus developed my skills in family therapy, developed a support program for women with babies under two months, and began to develop training programs for psychologists and social workers on how to use their family therapy skills with families from non-english speaking backgrounds with the then regional migrant health adviser Helen Boynton.

It was not long before I was seconded to work on new programs being developed, conducting sessions in the regional staff development area and working on projects related to building the skills of social workers working in regions with high numbers of people living in poverty. At a time when I was wondering whether I should specialise or keep learning and broadening my skills, I was advised by friends, 'you know what you can do and you know how to go back to it. You are a good clinician, community development worker and excellent group worker - go somewhere you don't know'.

So I moved into management, still in the outer western suburbs of Sydney, building community health services until an opportunity arose to participate at a director level in area health services with a subsequent secondment to conduct a review of an entire hospital and its communication processes from 'board level to the kitchen'. This was an opportunity where I learned a great deal about how hospital systems operate.

This led me to a similar role in an area health service which had high numbers of immigrant communities where the development of area health service policies, the evaluation of community health services, and the opportunity to contribute at board levels provided challenges and learning opportunities about management and communication. So when I was encouraged to apply for the position of director for the first torture and trauma rehabilitation service in Australia, I was told, 'you can do clinical work, you can do community work, you can do group work, you can do management, you can train people so apply'.

This was a wonderful opportunity to attend training programs held in Sydney where Dr Inge Genefke and Bent Sorenson from Copenhagen presented their work on developing the first torture and trauma service in the world, and to meet Professor Richard Mollica, then director of the Indo-Chinese Psychiatry clinic in Boston. I had ideas about how a similar service in Sydney could be developed, unique to an Australian context, with larger numbers of communities more widely spread than those in either Denmark or in Boston. Developing this service from a small grant with three FTE equivalent staff into (before I left 10 years later) an internationally recognised best practice model, facilitating the development of a similar service in each state in Australia securing a policy framework for refugee health in NSW, and engaging the organisation as the 4th collaboration centre with the World Federation of Mental Health - I had well and truly journeyed through twists and turns into a trauma field where I thrived.

This is the story of how I became and progressed as a trauma worker. As I mentioned earlier, there are many different trajectories that guide people onto the road to becoming a trauma worker and, more often than not, personal traumatic experiences in their pasts often shape their decisions. *Here are some examples of different trauma worker career paths:*

THE PLANNED CAREER

Brenda came from Africa and, as a psychologist, forged a planned career working in remote places around the world. Her work involved managing staff for international aid organisations in countries where human rights abuses were occurring. She worked away from her family following up new contracts for her services every few years.

After about 15 years she suddenly crashed. She knew herself she was suffering from Post-Traumatic Stress Disorder after witnessing atrocities. She took months off her work to establish a private practice and took up further study at an overseas university. People who work in most human rights organisations - particularly where human rights abuses are occurring - know they will be exposed in ways unlike other people. Their experience becomes more difficult when they find themselves dealing with managers whose behavior is not human rights sensitive, is unethical, or who bully their staff either subtly or openly thus adding a complex layer to the trauma workers' experience.

I remember attending a party in Sydney a little while after the outbreak of war in Bosnia. A young man at the party had recently returned to Australia after 12 months volunteering as a truck driver in Bosnia for an American-based International AID organisation. He was driving food trucks into dangerous areas and said 'every week one of my staff was killed.' It was clear he was feeling disconnected from what was happening around him and said he did not know what services could support him since his return to Australia. He said, 'the American staff got some support after but those of us from other countries didn't.'

Even though people may have a planned trajectory into working in trauma areas it does not mean they are immune to having flashbacks and nightmares about stories they have heard or events they have witnessed. Sometimes people can feel guilt at having survived fatal situations or at having a life back home so different to what they were exposed to in the field. Many of these are normal reactions. It can also be hard for people to leave the work they are doing to move on with other parts of their lives feeling a sense of responsibility to those they are leaving behind. Sometimes in these situations even managers of trauma organisations - especially those who have set them up - feel they are indispensable and stay for 20-30 years not recognising that sometimes organisations can be re-energised and revived through new management.

THE UNPLANNED CAREER

On the other hand, there can be a lack of stability due to the lack of funding and resources for those working in the trauma field. Richard works for a small faith-based humanitarian project and helps young people whose lives have been torn apart by migration and underemployment.

‘I hear horrific stories,’ he says. ‘Who else is going to help these kids or give them a chance? But it’s hard for us as well. There is no money for debriefing.’ Financial pressures obviously have an impact upon the organisation where the trauma workers help their clients and the opportunity to talk with someone about the impact of what they hear and see, while vital, is often unfunded. We have all experienced the health professional who does not seem connected with their job. They have lost any original passion they had. We can feel their sense of it being ‘just a job’. Compare that to the clinician who loves what they do. It is a different feel and experience. A 2014 article in The Guardian reported on a study on the levels of Post-Traumatic Stress Disorder in people who had worked in humanitarian fields where researchers discovered that around 30% had symptoms of PTSD after they returned home.

PTSD is now a recognised psychological condition. A number of symptoms group into several key areas where people may re-experience different things that happened to them; they may avoid reminders or become hypersensitive to sights, sounds, smells, taste, or feelings associated with what they experienced. It is not only aid workers who have emotional responses due to their workplaces. Student domains such as university campuses have in the past used abusive bastardisation (motting or hazing processes) to induct new members. These invariably had acts where physical and sexual abuse and humiliation were part of the process to ‘make them one of us’. Lenard, a senior health worker, commented, ‘I had nightmares for years and dropped out of the course after they did what they did to me. To this day I can’t even talk about it to anyone. I know I should but I’m afraid the nightmares will come back.’

THE ACCIDENTAL CAREER

When the 2004 tsunami and earthquake hit the Indonesian province of Aceh in December, hundreds of Indonesian students from Jakarta and people from Aceh became involved in helping the survivors and burying the dead. Over 200,000 people were killed in this international incident and over 800 non-government agencies descended on the capital Banda Aceh. Many of those who helped out had no previous experience of trauma work and with such a monumental humanitarian disaster there was little people could do but just keep on going. Many people stayed in trauma work after this event.

Some went on to contribute to international research on the after-effects of the tsunami. I had the opportunity to evaluate trauma services in Aceh six months after the tsunami and then 12 months after that. What became noticeable was the increase in jaded and exhausted staff. Some from the large international NGOs seemed emotionally remote as they managed their heavy workloads and high staff turnover. The restaurant supporting the recreational needs of the expat community was full on a Friday evening. As one person from a major international NGO said, 'this is where we come every Friday night so we can forget we are here in Aceh.'

THE CAREER CHOICE

I work with young professionals who early in their careers made the decision to work in trauma settings. They identify the courses they need to do and the organisations they need to work in to move to the settings they want. If they are fortunate they receive excellent guidance and supervision to facilitate their career trajectory – often able to take on postgraduate studies while working with trauma survivors. While managing the first torture and trauma service in Australia, the opportunity to take up postgraduate study provided a respite from stories of torture and enabled me to contribute to and develop research for that organisation, which substantially facilitated extra funding for it. This opportunity to study, develop projects, and initiate programs enabled a work balance that mitigated the effects of trauma stories not only for myself but for all the staff in the service at that time. Even when working in trauma as a career choice, it is important to build in the support and variety in roles to assist the energy and capacity to maintain the work.

THE ON-LINE TRAUMA WORK ENVIRONMENT

I include this as more and more organisations providing counselling and support are moving to the on-line environment such as telephone counselling or internet chat-type counselling environments. This can include people registering trauma stories for legal purposes such as victim support services, or after hours telephone and online counselling environments where counselling occurs over the phone or through written chat sessions between counsellors (trained or untrained) and specific client groups, or video counselling sessions. Many of these kinds of services are provided after-hours where there may be limited supervisory support than one would normally have in a day-to-day, face-to-face trauma service. I think these are unique contexts for trauma work and trauma workers. For untrained trauma workers taking information from clients in a call centre environment — pressures to limit call times while hearing trauma details, and short breaks for lunch and morning or afternoon tea — create particular stressors. It may be difficult for workers to shut off at the end of the day. Or they may become more and more remote in their client interactions, going through the motions, sometimes feeling a lack of achievement in their work. Trauma workers in this setting may need to ensure they have extra supervision and support. Many organisations organise a monthly support session with instructions from managers to come and talk to them at any time. This may or may not meet the needs of these telephone/on-line workers.

It is important these workers have in place some processes and/or rituals to assist them to leave their work behind. It can sometimes be as simple as making a conscious decision as you leave work, stepping across the threshold from your workplace to the outside world, to 'leave x, y, z, behind.' Other options include having an opportunity to tell someone what worked well that day and what you want to let go of. Even maintaining a journal with some of the above can provide a way of managing the extra stresses at the end of an on-line call shift. For many telephone/on-line trauma workers, a major challenge can be coping with the effects of short breaks and changing shift work patterns. Few on-line counselling agencies provide either stand-up desks or treadmill desks for their trauma workers. The effects on the physical health of these workers as they age are likely to include high blood pressure, heart disease, metabolic syndrome because, as we now know, the long-term effects of working in sedentary occupations are not ameliorated by weekend sessions at the gym.

KEY QUESTIONS TO ASK YOURSELF:

How did you get into trauma work?

How did this way of coming into trauma work impact upon you?

What would you do differently?

How will this affect your next career decision?

What work role variety is possible in your day to day work?

Chapter 8

How is trauma diagnosed?

People exposed to traumatic events often develop a wide range of symptoms. It is common for people to be assessed for PTSD or for complex trauma. There are a number of assessment scales that are used by psychiatrists, social workers, psychologists and counsellors to identify the range of traumatic events that their clients have been exposed to or specific symptoms that they may be experiencing. For trauma workers, the main scales available assess for secondary traumatic stress, compassion fatigue, vicarious trauma, burnout, and changes in cognition of the worker and their quality of life. Sometimes many of these terms are interchangeable; however they also have different meanings.

- Secondary traumatic stress occurs in trauma workers who work with trauma victims or survivors. The worker can begin to experience symptoms of post-traumatic stress or may begin to re-experience previous traumas they have had in their lives.
- Compassion fatigue refers to the ways in which trauma workers can become personally and emotionally depleted. These trauma workers can begin to become remote towards clients and may find it more and more difficult to engage in a positive way with them.
- Vicarious trauma refers to the changes that can occur in trauma workers' ways of thinking. They may begin to believe increasingly that the world is unsafe and behavioural changes occur in response to these different thought patterns and belief changes.

- Burnout is not exclusively linked to trauma workers. It can occur due to workplace stresses such as having too much to do in too little time. It presents in workers generally as emotional exhaustion.

The US-based National Child Traumatic Stress Network offers the following list of some of the symptoms that can occur for people working with trauma victims or survivors: (www.nctsn.org/resources/topics/secondary-traumatic-stress)

- Hypervigilance
- Hopelessness
- Guilt
- Avoidance
- Survival Coping
- Social Withdrawal
- Minimising
- Anger and /or Cynicism
- Sleeplessness
- Insensitivity to Violence
- Illness
- Fear
- Chronic Exhaustion
- Physical Ailments
- Disconnection
- Poor Boundaries
- Loss of Creativity
- Inability to Embrace Complexity
- Inability to Listen or Avoidance of Clients
- Diminished Self-Care

Sometimes these symptoms can become serious enough that people leave trauma work which is unfortunate since their skills are then lost to clients. While many trauma workers may have some symptoms on assessment scales, these are not always at clinically significant levels.

What is Post-Traumatic Stress Disorder (PTSD)?

Post-Traumatic Stress Disorder, or PTSD, is a series of symptoms that can develop after experiencing a traumatic event in which the person has concerns for their life. It is commonly known as a normal reaction to an abnormal event. People can develop a mixture of symptoms related to direct exposure to an event: intrusive symptoms of the event; and avoidance of reminders of the event.

Negative alterations in thoughts and mood and alterations in arousal and mood can also occur. Generally if these symptoms have been present for more than one month it may indicate PTSD.

The kinds of stressors that can lead to PTSD include: death; threatened death; actual or threatened serious illness; or actual or threatened sexual violence.

The most recent diagnostic criteria for identifying PTSD is in the Diagnostical Statistical Manual (DSM) Version 5 of the American Psychiatric Association. There are several criteria that need to be considered before diagnosing PTSD. Generally, symptoms need to have been present for about six months for a full diagnosis to be made.

Criterion A Stressor	The person was exposed to: death, threatened death, actual or threatened serious injury, or actual or threatened sexual violence.	**One** of the following events must be present: Direct exposure by witnessing, in person. Indirectly, by learning a close relative or close friend was exposed to trauma. If the event involved actual or threatened death, it must have been violent or accidental. Repeated or extreme indirect exposure to aversive details of the event(s), usually in the course of professional duties (e.g. first responders, collecting body parts, professionals repeatedly exposed to details of child abuse). This does not include indirect non–professional exposure through electronic media, television, movies, or pictures.
Criterion B Intrusion Symptoms	The traumatic event is persistently re–experienced.	**One required:** Recurrent, involuntary, and intrusive memories. NB: Children older than six years of age may express this symptom in repetitive play. Traumatic nightmares NB: Children may have frightening dreams without content related to the trauma(s). Dissociative reactions (e.g. flashbacks) which may occur on a continuum from brief episodes to complete loss of consciousness. NB: Children may re–enact the event in play. Intense or prolonged distress after exposure to traumatic reminders. Marked physiologic reactivity after exposure to trauma–related stimuli.
Criterion C Avoidance	Persistent effortful avoidance of distressing trauma–related stimuli after the event.	**One required:** Trauma–related thoughts or feelings. Trauma–related external reminders (e.g. people, places, conversations, activities, objects, or situations).

Criterion D Negative alterations in cognitions and mood	Negative alterations in cognitions and mood that began or worsened after the traumatic event.	**Two required:** Inability to recall key features of the traumatic event (usually dissociative amnesia; not due to head injury, alcohol, or drugs). Persistent (and often distorted) negative beliefs and expectations about oneself or the world (e.g. 'I am bad'. 'The world is completely dangerous'). Persistent distorted blame of self or others for causing the traumatic event or resulting consequences. Persistent negative trauma-related emotions (e.g. fear, horror, anger, guilt, shame). Markedly diminished interest in (pre-traumatic) significant activities. Feeling alienated from others (e.g. detachment or estrangement). Constricted affect: persistent inability to experience positive emotions.
Criterion E Alterations in arousal and reactivity	Trauma related alterations in arousal and reactivity that began or worsened after the traumatic event.	**Two required:** Irritable or aggressive behaviour Self-destructive or reckless behavior Hypervigilance Exaggerated startle response Problems with concentration Sleep disturbance
Criterion F Duration	Persistence of symptoms.	In criteria B, C, D, E for more than one month.
Criterion G Functional significance	Significant symptom-related distress or functional impairment.	Functional impairment (e.g. social, occupational).
Criterion H Exclusion	Disturbance is not due to medication, substance use, or other illness.	
Other notes	With dissociative symptoms.	In addition to meeting criteria for diagnosis, an individual can also experience high levels of either of the following as a reaction to trauma-related stimulus: De-personalisation — this is the experience of being an outside observer, a sense of being detached from one's self e.g. feeling as though something is not happening to you, or feeling like you are experiencing a dream. De-realisation — an experience of unreality, distance, or distortion... things are not experienced as real.

Complex trauma

People with long histories of trauma based on events in childhood are said to be experiencing complex trauma. Trauma histories that start in childhood and continued exposure to traumatic events throughout life characterise this kind of trauma.

Secondary traumatic stress

This summarises the kinds of symptoms that trauma workers can develop when working with traumatised clients. There are mixed views in the literature available about trauma workers and the development of secondary stress, with some studies disputing whether trauma workers frequently experience clinically significant levels of symptoms. Other studies indicate that up to 30% of aid workers returning to the UK after working in and witnessing human rights abuse do develop symptoms of post-traumatic stress. Further to that, some report that mental health workers who have personal trauma histories do often have higher levels of secondary traumatic stress.

Vicarious trauma

Vicarious trauma refers to the results for trauma workers of ongoing exposure to traumatic stories /experiences of other people. It is an indicator of the impact of trauma work on a trauma worker who may experience similar symptoms as their clients and over time it is generally regarded that this compromises the physical and mental health of the trauma worker. To manage it effectively, trauma workers who are also trauma survivors may need to be particularly vigilant in acknowledging their own needs, limits, emotions and resources. They may need to build into their lives effective ways of balancing the care they give to others with care they need to give to themselves.

This needs to include work/life balance. Self-care needs to become routine not only a once-in-a-while occurrence. Having a focus on connecting with others (not only clients who are trauma survivors) is important. I have seen many trauma workers limit their social contacts to other people who work in trauma fields, or in activist activities associated with the trauma survivor groups they work with.

While this may be something others find laudable, it does not lead to a very balanced lifestyle. The following is a list of the ways that vicarious trauma may manifest itself in the life of the trauma worker who is also a trauma survivor. Thinking about the ways that you can see this happening in your life can help you think about activities you may be able to implement as your personal prevention strategy against vicarious trauma, secondary stress and burnout.

Signs/Symptoms	Ways I notice this in me	Prevention activities I can put in place
Hypervigilance		
Suspicion of others		
Sleeping problems/ nightmares		
Intrusive images		
Anxiety		
Numbness		
Inability to experience pleasure		
Excessive care–giving (work and home)		
Cynicism		
Shame about no longer feeling warm, compassionate, optimistic		
Own issuers–activated		
Anger and irritability		
Fatigue and exhaustion		
Reduced tolerance for 'petty problems'		
Depression		
Self–criticism increased		
Estranged from others		
Challenges to own cognitive schema i.e. how you see the world		
Challenges about seeing the world as safe, just, controllable, and meaningful		
Feeling burdened by knowing terrible things that happen e.g. despair		
Examining life priorities – can be good – could be disruptive		

What is resilience?

Resilience involves being able to spring back into shape in some kind of way. Recent psychological literature suggests our biology and cultural heritage are loss and trauma-sensitive. In psychological and sociological literature, there are four key aspects to resilience:

1. People's ability to withstand negative results of stressful challenges;
2. Comparing groups of people who had different responses after a traumatic life event;
3. Ways people maintain commitment to important life tasks despite challenges; and
4. Assets that have a positive relationship and outcome after events.

Despite the different focus in each of these broad definitions it is clear that people have survived trauma in many ways throughout history. Similar to resilience, survivorship also focuses on the ways that people and groups adapt to trauma. Several factors seem to be helpful in promoting resilience after traumatic events. These include: developing a sense of safety, being able to stay calm, having a sense that one can get through the events, having connections to others and maintaining hope.

What is post-traumatic growth?

Post-traumatic growth refers to the adaptations that people can make to traumatic experiences that help their healing. It recognises that people can be distressed and can also grow from the experience and that these states can co-exist. Many people volunteer in services and areas related to their trauma as a positive contribution and a way of meaning-making from their experience. Some people write their trauma story, compose music, create artwork, plays or movies, and others participate in advocacy activities. Trauma workers might continue to work in areas related to traumas they have experienced or work in other areas of trauma.

As one worker said to me, 'trauma organisations have the highest numbers of people working in them who are trauma survivors themselves.' It has been proposed that up to 90% of trauma survivors report some positive changes following their trauma. As one man, an international management consultant who had two different chronic life-threatening cancers, said to me, *'I feel glad for them. They have changed me. I am a much more humble man.'*

Strengths that trauma workers who are trauma survivors bring to their work:

Trauma workers who are also trauma survivors can bring enormous strengths to their work and have identified a number of strengths that they believe can enhance their working relationships with their clients:

- Commitment – the quality of being dedicated to something/ someone or to stay on course with something you agree to do
- Compassion – having concern for the suffering of others
- Connection – linking with a situation or another person
- Deep empathy – ability to understand and share the feelings of someone else
- Determination – having a firm purpose to assist
- Engagement – making agreements to do something
- Experience – having directly acquired skills and knowledge
- Faith – having complete trust and confidence
- Healing – creating processes to become sound and healthy
- Hope – a feeling of expectation and desire for something to happen
- Inner knowing – having knowledge and awareness that only a few people have
- Recovery – a return to a normal state of health, mind or strength
- Resilience – being able to spring back into shape
- Resources – having materials, people, assets that can be drawn on; abilities to support one's self; being a source of help and information
- Skills – specific abilities
- Survival – being able to continue to live regardless of difficult circumstances
- Tenacity – being able to hold onto something firmly
- Tools – having something that helps to carry out a function
- Understanding – being consistently able to comprehend something

- Unique perspective - an individual view on situations and people
- Wisdom - quality of having experience and knowledge that can be drawn upon

As one trauma worker said, we bring a *'deep personal understanding of the wound to connection and the ongoing struggle to build connection'* and, as Joanne Fedler wrote in her novel *'Things Without a Name,'* the protagonist, Faith, a worker in a rape crisis centre, says:

> *Part of my job is to receive the horror, as though it were a changeling. And hold it just because it is human and I've been asked to. Someone's got to!. . . . I am doing Something Important and Useful. I am bearing witness to this injustice. (pages 17-19)*

KEY QUESTIONS TO ASK YOURSELF:

> What are the key strengths that you have developed through your trauma work or trauma experience(s)?
>
> What key strengths keep you working when organisational demands are the greatest?
>
> What key strengths do you have to call on when you feel overwhelmed by your trauma work?

Chapter 9

From trauma to thrives

A challenge for trauma workers who are traumas survivors is how to move from **Traumas to Thrives** in ways that enhance their work and personal lives**.** This too has relevance for managers of trauma workers who are trying to provide and expand services while maintaining staff morale and commitment. In the next sections we will look at some ideas about how this can be done.

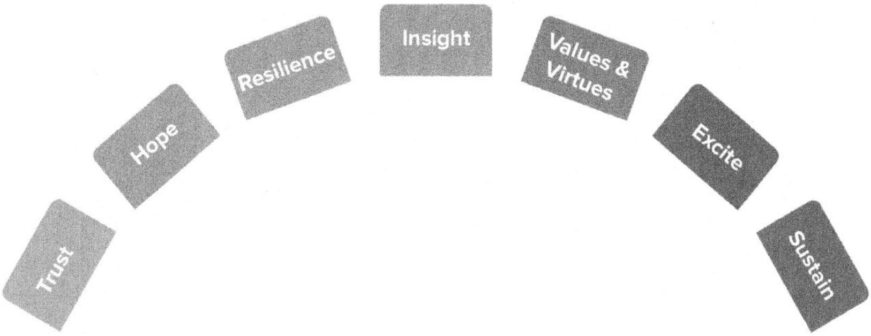

Trust

When we trust someone we believe in their reliability. We accept what they say and do without question. The experience of trauma can distort our ability to trust others and, more importantly, our ability to trust ourselves. I was reminded once by a midwife, *'trust your body, trust your baby, trust yourself.'* Knowing how to trust ourselves and our own bodies and our own inner being are necessary qualities for trauma workers.

Hope

When we want something to happen or we have the belief that something good can happen then we are experiencing hope. Hope has been defined as a positive state comprising success in having goal-directed energy as well as planning to meet goals. People who have experienced trauma may have periods of hopelessness. It may be useful for trauma workers to keep track of their hope levels using a scale such as the Trait Hope Scale developed by the social psychologist CR Snyder.

Directions

Read each item carefully. Using the scale shown below, please select the number that best describes YOU and put that number in the blank provided.

1. = Definitely False (DF)
2. = Mostly False (MF)
3. = Somewhat False (SF)
4. = Slightly False (SlF)
5. = Slightly True (SlT)
6. = Somewhat True (ST)
7. = Mostly True (MT)
8. = Definitely True (DT)

	DF	MF	SF	SIF	SIT	ST	MT	DT
1. I can think of many ways to get out of a jam								
2. I energetically pursue my goals								
3. I feel tired most of the time								
4. There are lots of ways around any problem								
5. I am easily downed in an argument								
6. I can think of many ways to get the things in life that are important to me								
7. I worry about my health								

	DF	MF	SF	SIF	SIT	ST	MT	DT
8. Even when others get discouraged I know I can find a way to solve the problem								
9. My past experiences have prepared me well for my future								
10. I've been pretty successful in life								
11. I usually find myself worrying about something								
12. I meet the goals I set for myself								

Scoring

a) The agency i.e. goal-directed energy subscale — add together items 2, 9, 10, and 12;

b) The pathway i.e. planning to meet goals subscale — add together items 1, 4, 6, and 8.

For the total Hope Scale score add together the totals for a) and b). The higher the scores the more hopeful: having goal-directed energy and a pathway to meet goals.

Resilience

If we are described as 'resilient', then people regard us as having the capacity to recover quickly from difficulties. We have an element of 'toughness' with regards to what we are able to overcome. Recent resilience literature emphasises a range of strategies for developing resilience.

In the book *'The Survivor Personality,'* Dr Al Siebert reminds us that *'life is not fair – and that can be for good for us.'* He describes empathy as a survival skill and discusses ways to turn misfortune into luck, discusses the importance of resources such as intuition, creativity and imagination, and encourages us to manage our healing and transform surviving into thriving.

Most models for building resilience include the importance of caring for one's self in a balanced way that includes physical exercise and activities that you find pleasurable.

Maintaining connections with others, accepting the life reality of change, participating in new activities and maintaining positive and hopeful outlooks all assist in building our resilience to what life throws at us.

Insight

The characteristic of insightfulness indicates the capacity to gain an accurate and deep understanding of someone or something. The person has an awareness that their mental experiences are not necessarily based on external realities.

Values and Virtues

Values are the principles or standards of behavior affecting one's judgements about what is important in life. It is important to know what one's key values are which can direct us in who we are and how we want to live. Virtues are qualities considered morally good or desirable in a person and their behavior can indicate a high (or low) moral standard. It is equally important to understand what virtues we want to develop in our own lives and in our relationships with others. To be clear about how we want to treat others and the ways we want to be treated. It can be easy for trauma workers to be more accepting of other's behavior than they receive themselves.

Excite

Having strong feelings of enthusiasm and eagerness. Having a state of increased energy or activity within the physical or biological system. Implementing strategies to ensure one's excitement about life and living is enhanced.

Sustain

Strengthen or support ourselves physically or mentally, despite bearing the weight we feel at times. Trauma workers need to sustain ourselves as well as others. In her poem *'The Journey,'* Mary Oliver gives an account of the journey taken by trauma workers who are also trauma survivors:

The Journey

One day you finally knew
what you had to do, and began,
though the voices around you
kept shouting
their bad advice--
though the whole house
began to tremble
and you felt the old tug
at your ankles.
"Mend my life!"
each voice cried.
But you didn't stop.
You knew what you had to do,
though the wind pried
with its stiff fingers
at the very foundations,
though their melancholy
was terrible.
It was already late
enough, and a wild night,
and the road full of fallen
branches and stones.
But little by little,
as you left their voices behind,
the stars began to burn
through the sheets of clouds,
and there was a new voice
which you slowly
recognized as your own,
that kept you company
as you strode deeper and deeper
into the world,
determined to do
the only thing you could do--
determined to save
the only life you could save.

Chapter 10

Tools for trauma workers

It is in determining to save our own life that we may find some of the following exercises useful:

The trauma worker's trauma history

Often as workers we may forget how many traumatic experiences we have been exposed to in our lives – at home and at work. Often we assume that we become more resilient the more traumas we experience but this is not always necessarily the case.

Our personal experiences can be green, red, or orange lights for us. That is, they can help us to understand more which aids connection and engagement with the trauma survivor (green light). It can be harmful for us and the client if their experience and ours becomes too enmeshed (red light) or it may be neither here nor there (orange light). Acknowledging and mapping our traumatic experiences for ourselves also helps when we are undertaking our own psychotherapy and/or supervision.

Exercise – The intergenerational trauma genogram

A genogram is a tool used in family therapy to assist counsellors and family therapists to understand the family system and identify potential dynamics. It is a family tree that contains further information in symbols and pictures. Draw your own family tree with your grandparents, parents, and their siblings. Also draw your own immediate family.

Record on it traumas experienced by each person and indicate which relationships are healthy, cut-off, conflictual, too close, toxic or enmeshed.

The trauma workers trauma timeline

It can be useful to develop your own trauma time-line. Think over your life and place on a line various traumatic experiences you have been exposed to. If this does not come readily to you, some people find it easier to go from the most recent to the most distant event. It is wisest to do this exercise at a time where you are not too vulnerable. Lighting a candle, burning incense, and playing some soothing music can help to alleviate worries and concerns. Just because you have experienced personal trauma does not mean you cannot function as a trauma worker; indeed it can sometimes mean the opposite. However, it is important for trauma workers who are trauma survivors themselves to work on their issues through their own therapy and/or supervision. This will help you to connect with clients without becoming overly distressed.

Exercise - Making a trauma timeline

Drawing your own trauma timeline can help you put a lot of experiences in your life into perspective. I find that when I do this with clients as well as with fellow workers, it gives them an opportunity to stand back and bear witness to their own strengths and survival. Sometimes it helps people to make connections between experiences they have had in the past and what they are living through now.

WW	Poverty	Violent Father	Witnessed death in car accident	Listening to violent abuse
5	8	6-20	35	38-40

The kaleidoscope of you

I love kaleidoscopes. Scottish scientist David Brewster invented the kaleidoscope in 1816 and ever since I received my first one at about six or seven years old, I have had an ongoing fascination with these beautiful implements. I would lie on a lounge pointing it at the light and see what new images even the minutest movement could effect.

I amused myself for hours with the drift of images I could create just from holding it to the light. I did not know at the time that the word kaleidoscope evolved from three Greek words (kalos; eidos; and scopios) meaning beautiful form watcher.

Later, as an adult, I collected kaleidoscopes and would give demonstrations to preschool and primary school children about all the different ways they are made. The first one I bought for myself as an adult was while I was in the USA. I loved the small coloured designs inside it. I had it for many years before my youngest daughter exclaimed, *'look mummy it's full of dinosaurs.'* And so it was. Tiny dinosaur shapes when held to the light reflected circles, diamonds and other shapes. Some of my kaleidoscopes are made of wood with paua shell from New Zealand. My favourite is made from Tasmanian Black-hearted Sassafras wood and the two discs inside it enclose Tasmanian wildflowers.

I began to use the kaleidoscope as a metaphor for healing with clients and groups many years ago. Despite the fragility of the materials and the apparent disconnection of whatever the elements are that are held to the light, from this, beauty emerges. It seems to me a fitting metaphor we can use with clients. Sometimes working with a client to develop images for their own kaleidoscope can help them to remember who they are beyond their trauma. Trauma workers can also find this useful.

I developed the image on the next page as an introductory slide when giving a presentation on long-term missing persons, including my personal experience of not seeing one of my children for (at that time) eight years following a visit to her father from which she never returned. That was a deeply traumatic time for me but defining myself with the following graphic helped me to realise that I did not have to be consumed by this trauma in the context of giving a presentation.

While I deeply missed my daughter (and still do) there are many parts of who I am; a social worker who is the mother of a missing daughter being only one part of who I am.

Kaleidoscope of me

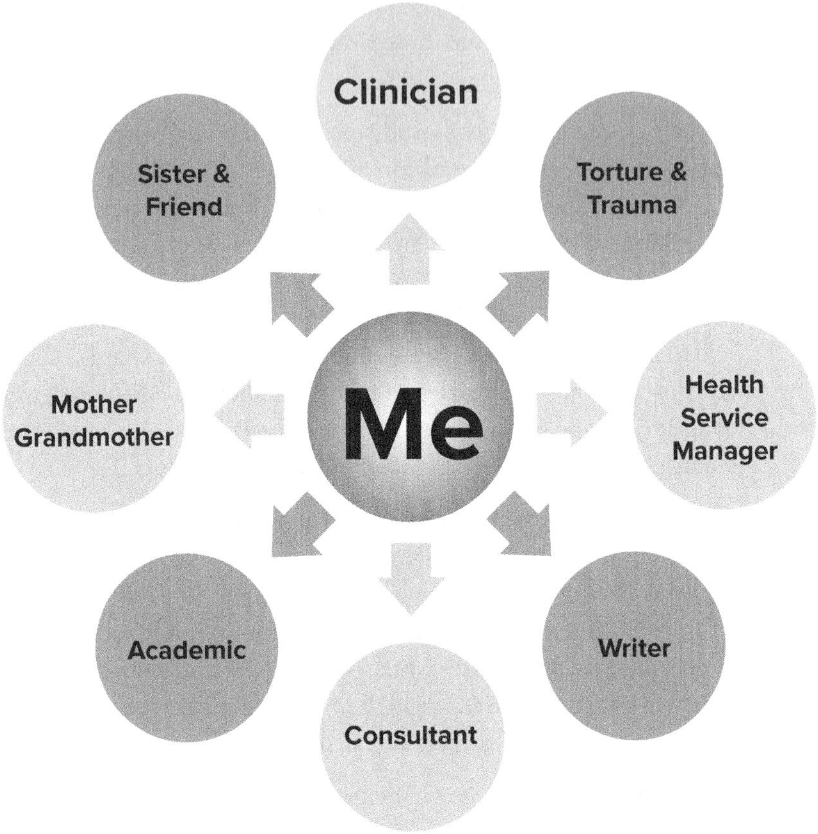

Exercise – Make a kaleidoscope as your personal healing tool

Kaleidoscopes can be simple structures to create. A round tube such as an empty toilet roll can be used. Decorate the roll with coloured paper on the outside.

Take a rectangle of silver foil long enough to fit inside the cardboard tube and fold it over lengthways to create a reflective surface. Create a peep-hole for the kaleidoscope by making a round disc with a hole in the centre and securing it to one end of the cardboard tube. Create a clear plastic cap the size of the other end of the tube. Fill this with small objects that inspire you – colours/stars/objects. You have now created something which you can keep on your desk and simply take a few deep breaths between clients and breathe in the beauty from your kaleidoscope.

(Instructions for making a kaleidoscope can also be found at inventors.about.com/od/lessonplans/ss/Kaleidoscope.htm) Alternatively you can, of course, purchase one.

I sometimes find a miniature kaleidoscope in my purse can provide me with a reminder of how colours and objects can be broken into beautiful shapes. There are also kaleidoscope apps for your mobile phone which allows us to bring some peace to our day regardless of the traumas we are witnessing, hearing, or living through.

Exercise - Strength mapping

Sometimes it is easy for trauma workers to forget the strengths they have. At least once a year, develop a visual image of your current strengths and strengths you wish to develop to assist you in moving forward in both your personal life and professional practice.

Your strength map can be a mind-map, a collage, written lists - however the more visual it is the easier it is to remind yourself of the gifts you contribute to others simply by being you. It can also be useful to divide up your strength map into the various areas of your life you currently have or wish to develop such as for home, friendships, relationships, spirituality, physical health, and work.

Exercise - The Circle of Life tool

The Circle of Life tool was developed in the Philippines while conducting a week long workshop in Tagatay with women from the Asia Pacific region who provided services to torture survivors while being torture survivors themselves. The workshop was funded collaboratively by the Danish AID agency DANEDA and Isis International, and brought together women from East Timor, Cambodia, Nepal, Bangladesh, Turkey, and the Philippines.

My colleagues and I used this exercise as a way to assist women to put their experiences into context while demonstrating a tool that they could use with their clients. The tool allows people to develop some perspective. It was featured in the book that we co-wrote at the end of the workshop called *'Recipes for Healing: Gender-Sensitive Care for Women Survivors of Torture.'*

Develop your own circle of life, based on the diagram below. Think of a traumatic experience that you had which still affects you today – then complete the questions in each of the quadrants to increase your understanding of the impacts and resources available to you.

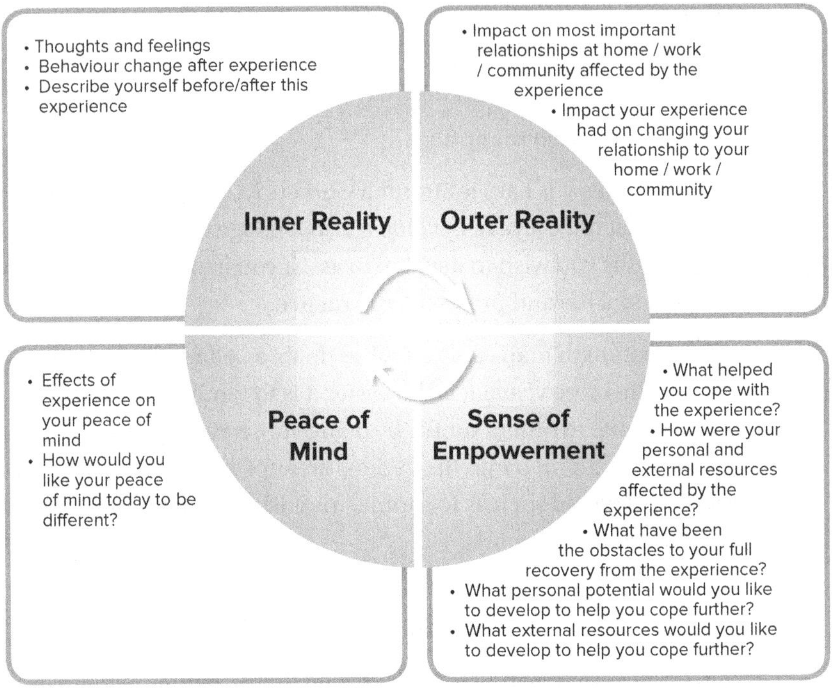

The Lotus tool

Whilst in the Philippines working with women who provided services to torture survivors, it became clear that many of the women in the group were trauma survivors themselves. After sharing our stories with one another as a group, we created the following symbol of our own healing and the key processes important to us to manage the events that had collectively occurred in our lives. The following diagram summarises the tools people used for healing:

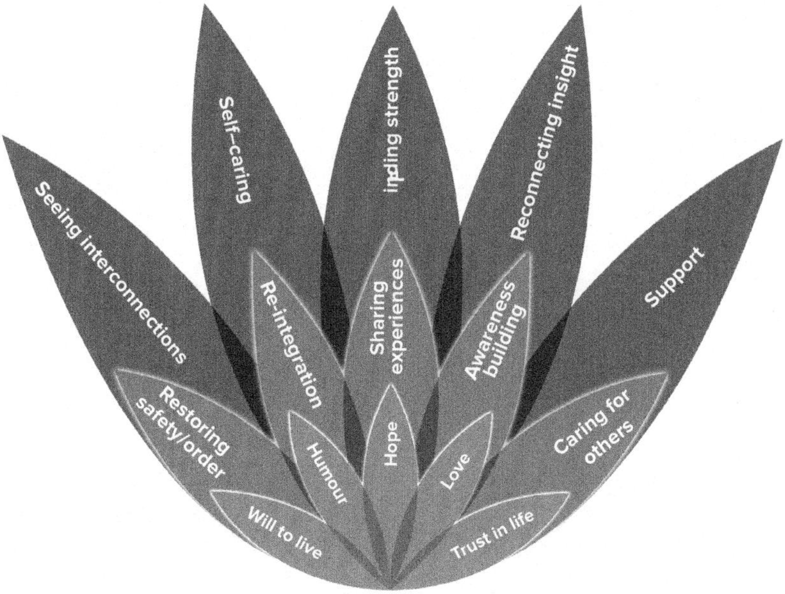

KEY QUESTIONS TO ASK YOURSELF:

Which exercise did you find most valuable for yourself?

Which one(s) could also be used with clients?

Chapter 11

How we cope

The Oxford English Dictionary defines coping as dealing effectively with something difficult. It is derived from a Middle English term meaning to 'meet in battle' or 'come to blows.' This is what it can feel like for the trauma worker who is also a trauma survivor – they have a sense of wariness about themselves and their coping abilities.

Invariably, they may fall into one of two camps in their workplace settings: there are those who are open about their past traumatic experiences and those who remain silent and rarely discuss it in the context of their work. Both positions can open up the trauma worker to criticism from peers and managers.

Either they are 'too open' and 'not contained' or are perceived as being distant and aloof. Frequently, when the trauma worker gets this kind of feedback, they are shocked as they do not link these behaviours to their own experiences of trauma and indeed they may not be related at all.

Generally we learn our coping skills in childhood through our role models in our families and communities.

However, for many trauma workers who are also trauma survivors, disrupted family and community experiences may mean they have underdeveloped and premature coping responses. *'I was three when I learned about hope,'* said one worker. *'It was many years later that I thought to myself, why would a three year old have to know about hope?'*

Functional coping skills

To function means to operate or perform and when we are coping well, we are able to face and deal with our responsibilities, problems, or difficulties. Inherent in ideas about coping is the pressure to perform, to battle on. For trauma workers who are also trauma survivors, this places an additional stress on them as they manage the trauma of their work lives along with the trauma of their own experiences. For example, we know that the anniversary of traumatic events can lead to a reliving or remembering of the experience. In trauma treatment processes people are encouraged to remember and talk about what happened to them and skillful clinicians know the importance of encouraging people to have greater self-care at the same time as balancing the influx of feelings and symptoms that can emerge.

Self-care is most effective when it is directed at our physical, mental, and emotional selves and we conduct it thoughtfully and mindfully rather than as a rote habit. It involves putting ourselves first especially in situations where it is not easy to have our normal supports with us, developing rituals of self-care can assist us to cope.

After the 2004 tsunami, I travelled through Aceh with a journal I was writing. At the end of each day I massaged some beautiful smelling lotion into my skin before I went to bed. This act of self-soothing connected me to myself and reminded me of my own strength. Journaling provided a way of putting the day to rest. I could write about what I saw and experienced and/or what had brought me joy in that day. (With my children, I would encourage them to tell me at the end of each day the things that had happened that they were 'glad about' and the things about themselves that they were 'glad about'.) Using these exercises in a situation where there was little support allowed me to keep myself connected to me.

Eating and sleeping

Trauma workers, whilst knowing the best ways to care for ourselves, frequently put others first and forget the simplest and most basic things which get us through the day. Couple this with times in our own lives when we may have extra stressors - such as caring for small children, caring for elderly or ill relatives, recovering from illness ourselves — and the consequences can be devastating.

It is therefore important to remind ourselves of the most simple and basic ways to practice self-care. We need to get back to basics: eat well, sleep well, drink lots of water, limit alcohol intake and get plenty of exercise.

Trauma workers sometimes have periods when sleeping well can become very challenging. This is particularly true after some intense casework, group work, or community work experiences. Winding down after work can develop into a vicious cycle of higher alcohol intake or medication to get to sleep, and a disturbed night's sleep once the alcohol or drugs wear off.

Alternatively, periods of insomnia can be interspersed with nightmares and dreams related to a client's stories or situations and/or your own experiences during the times they are trying to fall asleep. Engaging in sleep routines or obtaining advice and assistance from sleep experts or a general medical practitioner may help. Many people find exercise, yoga, relaxation music, watching comedies, being with animals and spending time in nature can all help.

KEY QUESTIONS TO ASK YOURSELF:

How would you describe your coping skills?

How balanced is your personal eating plan?

What changes could be made to improve your energy and ability to cope?

How much sleep do you have each day?

How functional and refreshing is it?

How can your sleep hygiene be improved?

Chapter 12

How trauma workers manage their challenges from trauma work

In my research on the key challenges trauma workers who are also trauma survivors face, there is a range of opinions and views. I have grouped their responses into main themes and summarised the ones people felt caused most pain and the reasons for this:

Potential barriers caused by their own traumas:

- Connecting and connectedness. As one worker said, *'I think connecting — when other people do not understand what you have gone through and the way it has affected you or do not just get it…[they] lack empathy'*
- Trusting others
- Maintaining hope
- Lack of in-depth case consultation
- Finding it difficult to listen to the experiences of others
- Creating/maintaining appropriate boundaries with clients
- How to respect others' perspectives on trauma that are radically different to our own — different values, different incorporations of the trauma
- Objectivity, where there is potential for being biased when dealing with cases
- Emotional responses to intervention

As one worker said, *'it would be most difficult to work with someone whilst trying to manage one's own feelings, especially if they had not yet been resolved.'*

Challenges related to re-living own traumas in their client work:

- Having to deal with their own past regularly – feelings from their own trauma surfacing; and dealing with constant reminders
- Working with the traumas of others on a regular basis – particularly when other people experienced the same traumas as the trauma worker
- Working with perpetrators of their own trauma
- Watching someone else suffer and having to help them
- Being triggered when working with clients; i.e. something their client says or does reminds them of themselves and/or something in their history
- Continuous exposure to the suffering of others
- Believing that what worked for them will work for others

As another worker said, *'unresolved personal trauma — because the trauma work is already so hard, and lack of attention to self-care can cause long term mental health (and health) problems. As caregivers, we have a hard time asking for help.'*

Challenges due to not being aware of impact of trauma:

- High level of countertransference and the energy it takes to attend to it
- Own unresolved trauma
- Becoming too attached
- Overstepping professional boundaries
- Normalising things through their own experience rather than the clients
- Managing their own trauma
- Development of vicarious trauma
- Projecting own trauma into presenting cases
- Understanding how to learn from our experience of trauma without imposing our learning on others
- Understanding that our work is about our healing others without utilising their pain to help our own healing

- Questioning their own competence: is the worker there because they fulfil the requirements/competencies, or because of having personal experience with that trauma?
- Separating their story from the story of others

Impacts for trauma workers related to outside their workplace:

- Inability to leave work at work
- Developing Post-Traumatic Stress Disorder
- Managing work/life balance
- Managing self-care
- Burnout
- Finding or creating a structure to care for oneself through non-judgmental supervision and consultation
- Fatigue
- Emotional drain
- Questioning/over thinking/personalising things in their personal lives

> A worker commented, *'of course, it depends on the person's own healing, but I think the continuous exposure to trauma can be the most painful. The toll this takes on someone is enormous and can undermine one's sense of the world being a safe place. Without a sense of safety and hope for all people in the future, it can be incredibly difficult to sustain a career in trauma work.'*

What are the strategies used by trauma workers who are also trauma survivors?

Trauma workers are a varied and eclectic group of people who have many ideas for strategies to manage the personal and organisational challenges in their work.

The table on the following page summarises responses from trauma workers.

Strategies for overcoming challenges faced by your trauma work experiences:

Focus Area	Challenge	Strategy
Personal	Own experiences	Re–visit the past in personal counselling sessions and understand what the ongoing impact of your trauma experience might be
	Identify personal challenges	Develop goals to overcome and move beyond them – self–reflection assists with this
	Past life situations	Understand you don't have to reside in your old life – change your life
	Resolving own trauma	Personal psychotherapy to manage own emotional response to personal trauma
	Creativity	Share own stories, create music, write, have a healthy self through the arts
	Creating safety	Imagery work/meditation to imagine safe healing spaces available to you
Relationships	Connections	Risk building new relationships Develop a support network
	Building trust	Be vulnerable and resilient
Work/Life	Being consumed by others' stories	Develop good work/life balance
	Taking work home	De–brief with a colleague at the end of the day or after a session with a client where you were triggered
	Collegiate relationships	Participate in group therapy with other trauma workers
	Know your triggers	Develop strategies to manage during and after client work
	Understanding effect of personal trauma on your work	Supervision with trusted and skillful supervisor/professional
	Creating meaning	Participate in advocacy activities to balance individual work with clients
	Having a life outside	Do not check work emails or phone calls during non–work periods such as weekends
	Reduce the impact of others' trauma on you	Develop varied work program – face to face work with clients plus some research, marketing, or development projects, or training and professional development activities

Focus Area	Challenge	Strategy
Self-care	Fatigue	Take time out when needed Physical breaks – such as holidays
	Developing a self–care plan	Write it down and diarise activities that cover both physical and mental strategies
	Maintaining health and fitness	Do some body work – dance, massage, exercise, sports Participate in social activities based on physical activity
	Learning one's limits	Recognise we cannot be all things to all people
Transpersonal	Maintaining faith	Develop a spiritual or meditation practice
	Reflection and meaning	Create space for meditation/prayer

Consider the following statements from experienced trauma workers:

There is a very fine line between a trauma survivor's ability to successfully and unsuccessfully help others trauma survivors. The worker (having survived trauma) needs to be extremely self-aware and constantly reflective to ensure their own experiences don't negatively impact themselves or their clients in any way.

I think that personal loss and trauma has allowed me to have more patience and trust in the process, and to truly understand the depth of another's pain. It isn't an abstraction. So now when someone says, "I feel this" I can say to myself, "I know what you mean." And I have trust in the power of healing from relationships, etc. You grow your capacity to sit with the pain before rushing to fix it.

KEY QUESTIONS TO ASK YOURSELF:

Which of the above quotes do you relate to and why?

What self-care activities can you implement to balance the traumas from your trauma worker experiences?

Chapter 13

Bridging our strengths to strengthen our living

When trauma workers who are trauma survivors speak about their lives, they name qualities such as resilience, experience, empowerment, motivation to change and move forward as key strengths. They may describe themselves as the *'wounded healer'* or, as one worker said, *'a person who has experienced trauma and through establishment of a therapeutic relationship has corrective experiences that can be created with other survivors.'*

They see their own personal experiences as understanding the complexities in self-disclosure and believe they are role models for their clients in living life after trauma. They have empathy and understand and know the path of healing in deep ways.

They believe they have a greater understanding of the challenges trauma victims have faced and through their own personal experiences have some knowledge of the strategies which may help with trauma symptoms. They have a deep knowledge of what trauma survivors experience and how unstable one's identity can be after a trauma(s).

They also have first-hand experience of survival and healing (hopefully) and can apply some of their personal tools and skills to their work. They often have a true understanding of the survivor experience and a deep and personal understanding of the wound to connectedness and the ongoing struggle to build connections. They believe they bring to their work faith, hope and wisdom. They commit to bearing witness to people's stories and bearing witness to those stories is an important part of their work with clients.

As one worker wrote to me:

> *We address the existential aspects of traumatic events through the storyteller–listener relationship and the manner in which this encounter opens up the possibility of the unknown — all dialogue has the potential for future friendship and affection but also for disappointment and conflict and, as therapist, having the courage to accept a promising but unpredictable outcome.*

In my individual and supervision groups with trauma workers they often identify several behaviours they build into their lives:

Keep humour in your life

Numerous research studies have been done on humour as a healing and preventive health practice. It can be easy to become weighed down by one's own issues in addition to those related to work and traumatised clients.

Many years ago, the 'modern father of laughter therapy' Norman Cousins used laughter as a healing tool and decided to spend a lot of time watching old comedy movies.

Subsequently, his illness left him and he wrote about his experiences in his book '*Anatomy of an Illness*.'

It is unclear exactly why humour works; however I suggest the following:

- Emotional release;
- Increases the circulation of 'feel good' hormones such as serotonin and dopamine;
- Often triggers laughter in others so there is a sense of companionship in the experience; and
- Reduces pain through the increase of endorphins, and reduces stress levels in the body.

I have seen people in a trauma response laugh uncontrollably while talking about some aspects of it. This is a stress release function which often assists the person to talk about their experience without totally falling apart.

The benefits of laughter

www.helpguide.org/life/humor_laughter_health.htm

Physical Health Benefits	Mental Health Benefits	Social Benefits
Boost immunity	Adds joy and zest to life	Strengthens relationships
Lowers stress hormones	Eases anxiety and fear	Atracts others to us
Decreases pain	Relieves stress	Enhances teamwork
Relaxes your muscles	Improves mood	Helps defuse conflict
Prevents heart disease	Enhances resilience	Promotes group bonding

There are many ways to bring humour back into your life. Make a commitment to only watch serious documentaries in work related contexts - not at home. Watch comedies at home instead, as Norman Cousins did. Remember things you did as a child that gave you pleasure and do some of those. As the saying goes *'it is never too late to have a happy childhood.'*

Treat the small child inside of you — blow bubbles with a bubble wand outside a supermarket if you want. This was something I did once, much to the embarrassment of my own children at the time and to the delight of everyone else's children. When I arrive home at the end of the day I am faced with a black cat given to me by one of my daughters, and a crazy and delightful dog, a Moodle or Maltipoo (Maltese cross Poodle) who delights me with his antics racing around the house, picking up toys, throwing them in the air, jumping over the cat, welcoming me with his 'glad you are home' routine that definitely makes me laugh. Yes, pets can bring us laughter.

Arts and crafts and other mindful pleasures

Anything that absorbs your mind and provides relief from trauma is helpful. For me it can take the shape of guitar playing, crocheting, or cross-stitching. Many hospitals and health centres incorporate art activities into their healing programs. After the tsunami in Aceh, the provision of art materials and the development of art and craft programs and other art forms provided ways in which people could transform their fears and concerns and record what the experience was like for themselves. Musical instruments were created from floating pieces of wood and metal. Drums were used to beat out the pain people felt. Singing groups in the community provided people with connection and hope.

Creating a healing garden

In 2002, Annalisa Gartmann Vapaa completed her Masters degree in Landscape Architecture on the defining characteristics of a healing garden. Her work focusses on different types of healing gardens: those used specifically for healing, those used for meditation, and those used to create a sense of sanctuary. She reminds us that gardens used for healing is not a new concept when one looks at some of the gardens associated with medieval buildings such as cathedrals and monasteries. She proposes that healing gardens for whatever purpose incorporate a number of attributes. They should:

- Appeal to the senses;
- Be easy to understand, navigate and use;
- Encourage wildlife;
- Provide seasonal change; and
- Promote reflection and provide relief from stress.

Most importantly it should be designed for the person who uses it. She recommends reflecting on colours and shapes and landforms you enjoyed as a child or an adult that give a sense of peace as one way of starting a healing garden for yourself. http://scholar.lib.vt.edu/theses/available/etd-05132002-115528/unrestricted/Healing_Gardens_Thesis_Vapaa.PDF

After my daughter went missing and many years of not knowing where she was, I came across some ceramics she had made as a child. From these I created a small garden, less than a metre squared, that comprised of some plants, her art, art belonging to other children no longer living with me, and symbols of loved ones who are no longer alive. When I look at this small space in my garden I am reminded of those I care about and those I still send love to whether they are with me or not. It is a place where I can cry if I wish to but more often than not it also provides a place representing me, my mothering, my strengths, as well as those of people close to me.

Building and maintaining relationships

It can be easy to keep putting work and clients before key relationships in our lives. Yet building and maintaining the relationships that nurture us is vital for trauma workers. These relationships can be with our spouses, significant others, our children, parents, other relatives, friends and neighbours.

Building and maintaining relationships takes time and commitment. Review your weekly schedule and schedule time to see people who provide you with support in your life. This is a perfect opportunity to combine an activity that you find nourishing with someone special to build and maintain those important relationships.

Keeping your spirit alive

What brings you awe? What inspires you to do great things and be greater than you are? Whatever these places, people, and activities are for you, these are the things that can keep you alive. Some people find religious activities part of this, others find meditation a way of finding inner peace, and for others activities such as sailing, surfing, bush-walking, or paragliding provide ways of seeing the world as bigger than themselves.

Virtues can help

According to the Oxford English Dictionary a virtue is 'behaviour showing high moral standards; or qualities desirable in a person.' While we often focus on understanding our values as important for enhancing and directing our lives, being able to also practice virtues which are meaningful to you can enhance both personal and professional relationships. The Virtues Project (www.virtuesproject.com) was developed in 1991 and defines 52 virtues synthesised from a wide range of philosophical and spiritual beliefs and backgrounds.

It covers 100 virtues which can be referred to individually, and used personally, or in family or educational settings. An adjunct to the project is the availability of cards which gives a summary for the meaning of each virtue and ideas for implementing it in one's life. While many of us focus on our values it is equally important to know and refer to our virtues. Our virtues assist in developing our character and our communications with others.

Some more strategies to keep yourself alive:

During the course of one year, I had been through several traumatic experiences while working in the field of missing persons.

Some of the people I spoke to had ongoing traumas related to the disappearance of a family member. For some it was a child, for others it was a mother, a sister, a parent, a grandparent or a friend. My mother had recently had a stroke and I was coordinating the contact with other family members. She subsequently died some weeks after her stroke leaving me with the major task of sorting out the house she and my father had lived in since the early 1970s. 'Over 30 years of pack-ratting,' I remarked to a colleague. It was during this time my sister, Sarah, now a union activist and teacher/librarian in a high school, sent me what I later called 'Sarah's Wisdom 4 Me'. I share this with you because sometimes as trauma workers we need a list just to remind us of what ways we can nurture ourselves:

- Listen to a favourite CD
- Watch a movie - preferably a comedy
- Have a treat - such as your favourite meal or snack - even better if it's healthy
- Relax in a bubble bath
- Buy some inexpensive candles and float them in a bowl where you can see it easily
- Burn your favourite incense (a particular favourite of mine is Nag Champa)
- Remind yourself - you have learned the gift of compassion, you demonstrate it to others often - now give it to yourself in abundance
- Colour in a picture
- Renovate your space - one small area at a time
- Select an inspiring or spiritual book and read a section each day

'Hold your own hand and give yourself what you did not receive from other,' my sister reminded me.

Further strategies:

- **Physical** - Massage; comforting touch; playful activities; healing/ sacred place at home and in office; radical self-care; simple pleasures

- **Psychological** - sharing feelings; venting emotions in safe ways; visualise or have a safe and nurturing place to visit regularly; journal writing (rapid writing); affirmations that counter negative thinking; have realistic expectations of self and others

- **Social** - social activities; try new things; get a friend to just listen for 15 minutes; clubs and other support organisations including religious groups

- **Spiritual** - reminder *'I didn't cause it, I can't change it, and I can't control it'*; engage in a spiritual practice that supports you; create rituals that have meaning for you; walk in nature; read inspirational materials; have inspirational quotes/images around you

Chapter 14

Professional sources of support

Supervision, Employee Assistance Programs & Therapy

In earlier chapters I identified some ways that trauma work impacts upon trauma workers. I will now look at some of the ways that trauma workers should utilise additional support.

Supervision

Most trauma workers, irrespective of their professional training, undertake supervision. This may be due to requirements from their agency, their professional associations or for their own self-development. In the following section on supervision I address many of the questions I am asked by supervisees about supervision.

The role of supervision

In many ways the choices to be made in selecting a supervisor can be similar to the experience that clients go through when choosing a counsellor:

- Finding the right person with the right skills
- Assessing your needs
- Organising mutually agreeable times to meet
- Deciding on frequency
- Developing a payment structure

Why should I have a supervisor?

Supervision is a professional relationship to assist you to grow and develop your clinical and personal skills in line with evidence-based practice and the code of ethics of your organisation. For counsellors, psychologists, social workers, occupational therapists and a host of other disciplines, supervision is an integral part of your continuing professional development and is increasingly becoming a requirement in order to belong to your professional association.

What is supervision?

In the counselling professions — whether you are a qualified social worker, psychologist, psychotherapist, counsellor, or whether you see clients through other models such as voluntary or ministerial — supervision is a process to ensure ongoing professional development and the maintenance of professional integrity.

Why is it important?

Supervision is important for a number of reasons. It:

- improves your professional credibility;
- provides professional support and another 'head' to think through challenging client or group situations;
- provides personal support for you as a developing practitioner — particularly in balancing professional and personal identities; and
- increases personal and professional self- knowledge.

Is it confidential?

This can depend on the nature of how you engage a supervisor. Some organisations have agreements with supervisors they fund for their staff which may impose limits on confidentiality such as if code of ethics has been breached.

As most supervisors represent professional disciplines with their own code of ethics, they may also have mandatory reporting guidelines should you disclose self-harm, potential harm to others, breaches in professional practice, and ethical dilemmas.

However for most supervision relationships, professional confidentiality is upheld and most supervisors will inform you of their confidentiality arrangements early in your supervisory relationship.

Does my supervisor have to work in the same field as me?

This depends on what you want from supervision. For some people it is important to them to know their supervisor has worked in the same contexts and understands their challenges from specific clinical settings. However, this is not always necessary.

Most people seek supervisors who can add to their clinical knowledge, skills and experience for their current position and/or for their future roles.

Is supervision the same as having an Employee Assistance Program?

Employee Assistance Programs are provided as part of Workplace Health and Safety programs. They are generally short-term relationships and focus on areas of personal difficulties as well as some workplace concerns such as relationships at work. Supervision is about your development as a skilled, ethical practitioner and your commitment to ensuring the best practice for your clients.

I am a new graduate and work in a trauma field

Supervision is particularly important during your first few years as a practitioner. It is during this time that you are learning how to apply your theoretical knowledge and frameworks to real life situations with clients, peers and colleagues. You may find the people you work with have less theoretical knowledge than you and it can feel disheartening to realise you are constantly seen as 'new' and 'young'.

Supervision can help you to make sense of how to integrate your theory and knowledge into the practical settings in which you now work. It can also provide a space to reflect on the impact of organisational cultures on you and your clients. It provides opportunities to begin to develop your career direction and plan your continuing professional development.

I am already a skilled and experienced trauma clinician

Supervision has probably been a key to your ongoing success and development. You may have had supervision experiences that have been beneficial as well as some which were challenging for a range of reasons. Supervision can continue to assist your personal and professional growth. It can engage you in career change and development. Many senior practitioners are invariably offered opportunities to move into team leading and management roles.

While many of our clinical skills are transferable to other work roles, supervision can assist you with the transition from clinician to manager, to senior executive. Taking this professional leap can be daunting as well as exciting.

Should my supervisor get supervision too?

Most supervisors will have their own professional supervision arrangements. This ensures their practice is current and relevant both in their field as well as in their supervision skills. It enables then to keep 'in tune' with the experience for supervisees of attending supervision. Many supervisors also do specific training to become more skilled as supervisors through their professional associations or through specific training providers.

What are the different ways supervision can be provided?

Many people opt for individual supervision. This is a one to one relationship through which trust and skills are built. Supervision can be provided to a group of social workers at the same time in an organisation. Sometimes supervision is provided internally in an organisation with more junior clinicians supervised by senior clinicians.

This can work very well however it can have drawbacks if there are personality clashes or when there is a need for the less skilled clinician to grow into senior roles. Supervision can also be provided through online means such as by skype, telephone, or other online contexts. Skype supervision is particularly valuable for clinicians in remote areas or in other countries.

My work provides me with a supervisor

Some trauma organisations fund professional supervision by an external supervisor for their trauma workers. This is either for individual or group supervision with other people you work with. It can be provided internally such as by another clinician in the organisation who is seconded to provide supervision or it may be externally with someone unrelated to the organisation. There are pros and cons to each system. An internal supervisor may have a close understanding of the organisational culture while an external supervisor may be able to give fresh perspectives from other areas outside the organisation.

Group supervision may be more threatening for trauma workers who are also trauma survivors with people feeling unwilling to disclose issues from their past. Group supervision is not a therapy group. It is designed to give people a reflective space to think and learn about their own practice. In some organisations the manager insists on participating in the group as *'they are a group member too and need supervision.'* However generally it is recommended that staff have an opportunity to discuss issues independently and discreetly.

What if my work won't pay for it?

Most professional associations in psychology, social work, occupational therapy, counselling and so on can provide information about supervisors. It can be recorded as a work expense for your income tax purposes particularly if you can obtain a support letter from your manager.

How do I know if my supervisor is good or not?

The best option is to ask around. However remember your response to someone may be different to another person. It helps if you have some idea about the kind of skills you want your supervisor to have.

Does it have to be done in person?

It is best if it can be done in person — however skype-based supervision or other technology that allows people to see each other in 'real time' can also be effective.

For people in rural areas this can be a suitable alternative and can also include group supervision through internet conferencing solutions.

What experience should I look for?

This question can be a little like 'how long is a piece of string?' You may want a supervisor who has worked in similar area as you with similar clients, or someone who has some of the skills you want to acquire; or someone who has a specific supervision or counselling methodology that you admire.

What qualities should I look for?

In my view someone you can get on with, who demonstrates dignity towards you, an effective listener who is able to challenge you to develop. These elements provide a suitable container for developing your supervisor-supervisee relationship. It is also important your supervisor is willing to ensure your psychological safety and is committed to assisting you to obtain help if you or anyone close to you is at risk of harm.

What is the cost?

This depends on the experience and qualifications of the person you are seeing. Costs can vary between $100–300 per session. You may be able to claim this on your income tax at the end of each year which means it is accepted as a work expense and reduces your taxable income. Check with your accountant or the taxation department about this.

How often do I need to attend?

Generally supervision occurs on a monthly basis. Though there have been instances where fortnightly supervision is held when people are working in highly traumatising contexts or due to unusual circumstances.

How do I find a supervisor?

Most professional organisations have databases of people who are available. Many of the people on these databases see clients as well as providing supervision services. Asking other professional people you know who they would recommend can also be useful. Approaching people directly who may have taught you, or whose work you have read, may also assist as well.

Note: *It is always important to remember that supervision is a professional mentoring /education relationship not necessarily individual counselling.*

Employee Assistance Programs

Employee Assistance Programs (EAPs) that are made available to staff are generally outsourced to organisations specialising in this work. Generally a company contracts one of these organisations to provide services to their staff primarily to complement Human Resources Departments. This ensures that staff has access to counselling support for situations affecting their health and wellbeing that could interfere with their work performance. It is one way that organisations can show how to value their staff.

Generally people who work as counsellors in EAPs are psychologists, counsellors, and social workers, many with postgraduate qualifications. However they generally only provide short-term counselling options of about six to 10 sessions. Services for EAPs are usually free to the client as they are borne by the company. Sessions are confidential however as with most clinicians in any service, there are mandatory reports meaning that should you or someone else be at risk of harm then counsellors may intervene with referral to emergency services.

For trauma workers who are trauma survivors, EAPs may be quite limiting if there are significant issues they wish to discuss where personal issues and their trauma work are intersecting. For example, when one of my children was taken in a parental abduction, the five sessions with my EAP counsellor focused on looking after myself: *'Dance more,'* the counsellor would say each week.

While I did and do enjoy dancing, when I decided to choose a different supervisor who was also a clinician and the result was a supervisor who was prepared to be there and witness the suffering I had at the time as well as discussing ways to look after myself without impacting on my work role at the time.

Therapy

Ensuring you are in the best psychological shape to do the work you do is especially important in trauma work. We do not know what and how we may be triggered in our work. Having a strong understanding of yourself can be helped by being willing to have therapy to address your own life experiences and traumas you have been exposed to. My first foray into counseling and therapy as a client occurred after the breakdown of my marriage which led to me and my two young children (aged four and six) living alone in a new area we had moved to as a family only six months previously.

Maintaining the mortgage for our home at the time meant living from pay to pay as the mortgage alone took 70% of my salary. I had married very young (21) virtually moving from my parents' home into a marriage with my first boyfriend. I had spent years supporting him as a student during the marriage and it was no surprise when the marriage ended. We had both been too young and in many ways were not suited to one another. So, left on my own with two small children, therapy focused on many aspects of my life prior to marriage and the choices I had made.

Since then I have been in therapy on many occasions - often with therapists with diverse styles and backgrounds. This assisted me to manage a partner who was emotionally abusive, issues around my childrens' adolescence, and helped me to address the impact of trauma work on myself and my family. I have been exposed to Jungian therapy, psychodynamic psychotherapy, somatic psychotherapy, process-oriented psychotherapy, and have experienced this as a gift that has maintained my passion and clarity for trauma work.

I have participated in a range of body-related therapies such as acupuncture, herbalism, Reiki, spiritual development, and kahuna training and bodywork. These have assisted me to understand the connections between my body and life experiences. Finding the right therapist (like finding the right supervisor) requires you to search out the kinds of processes and programs you believe may be beneficial for you.

Designing the right support networks for yourself

What is a support network? We may often think our friends and families are our only support networks. While they are important in our lives and can provide balance to our lives, it is important to also think through a range of support frameworks when we are trauma workers. Planning our approach to having support can go beyond addressing the ideas earlier about managing vicarious trauma. One of the strategies I built into my own management of trauma was recognising I needed to have one week away from work every three months rather than taking my three to four week holiday in one hit each year. Other people may find it more effective to have the longer break. In her book 'Life Makeovers', Cheryl Richardson recommends asking ourselves the following questions to help identify ways relationships are/are not supportive for us:

- Do you feel accepted for who you are?
- Are you judged and criticised unnecessarily?
- Do you receive as much from the person as you put in?
- Do you feel more energised after seeing this person?
- Do their values align with yours?
- Do they celebrate your successes with you? And importantly;
- How do you feel about yourself when you are with this person/people?

Chapter 15

A word to managers of trauma workers

When establishing the first treatment and rehabilitation service for torture survivors in Australia, we spent significant time as a group talking about the kind of culture we would have in this fledgling organisation. What were the principles and practices we would engender and what were the behaviours clients and other staff would see? How would our clients actually **know** we were both a human rights and a multicultural organisation – what would they be able to see, touch, smell, taste and feel? The reason we did this was to minimise the development of 'Parallel Process'. At the time, most of the staff had been torture survivors themselves and had been exposed to a wide range of human rights abuses. I reflected that some of the behaviours that could trigger abuse for them was in the style of management they experienced.

- Rules that did not make sense
- Having no choice about their work patterns
- Keeping information away from them
- Inadequate resources to work with
- Long hours in the same role
- Lack of recognition and acknowledgement
- Divide and rule management styles

If clients were to have a good experience with us then our staff needed to be managed in the way I expected clients to be addressed – with choice, freedom, and dignity, and a keen awareness of the potential impact of human rights abuse. Parallel Process means what happens for clients can become reflected in the staff system.

It acknowledges that when two or more systems interact - whether individuals, groups, organisations, or a network of organisations — issues between them are at risk of being continually acted out. When traumatised clients, stressed staff, and pressured organisations interact, then it is easy for the emotions that clients feel to become reflected at various levels in the organisations. It can lead to organisational behaviour impacting negatively on staff and clients, leading to increased organisational stress and may change some of the ways managers manage the service. In other words a vicious cycle occurs:

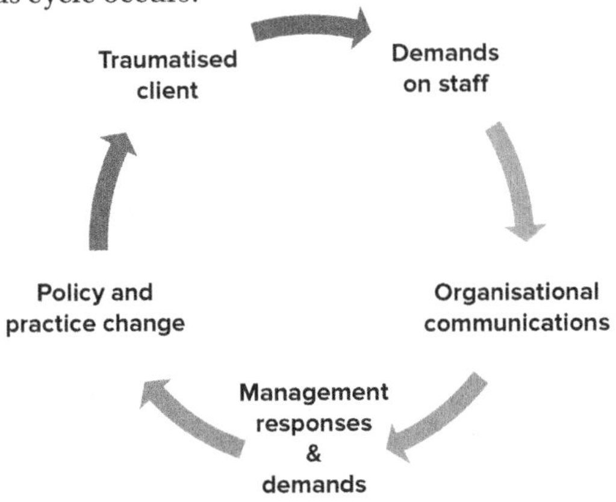

As one organisation states,

> *Leaders become variously perplexed, overwhelmed, ineffective, authoritarian, or avoidant as they struggle to satisfy the demands of their superiors, to control their subordinates, and to protect their clients. When professional staff and non-professionally trained staff gather together in an attempt to formulate an approach to complex problems they are not on the same page. They share no common theoretical framework that informs problem-solving. Without a shared way of understanding the problem, what passes as treatment may be little more than labelling, the prescription of medication, and behavioural "management". When troubled clients fail to respond to these measures, they are labelled again, given more diagnoses and termed "resistant to treatment". In this way, our systems inadvertently but frequently recapitulate the very experiences that have proven to be so toxic for the people we are supposed to help.*

The following graphic from Bloom and Farragher demonstrates this interplay:

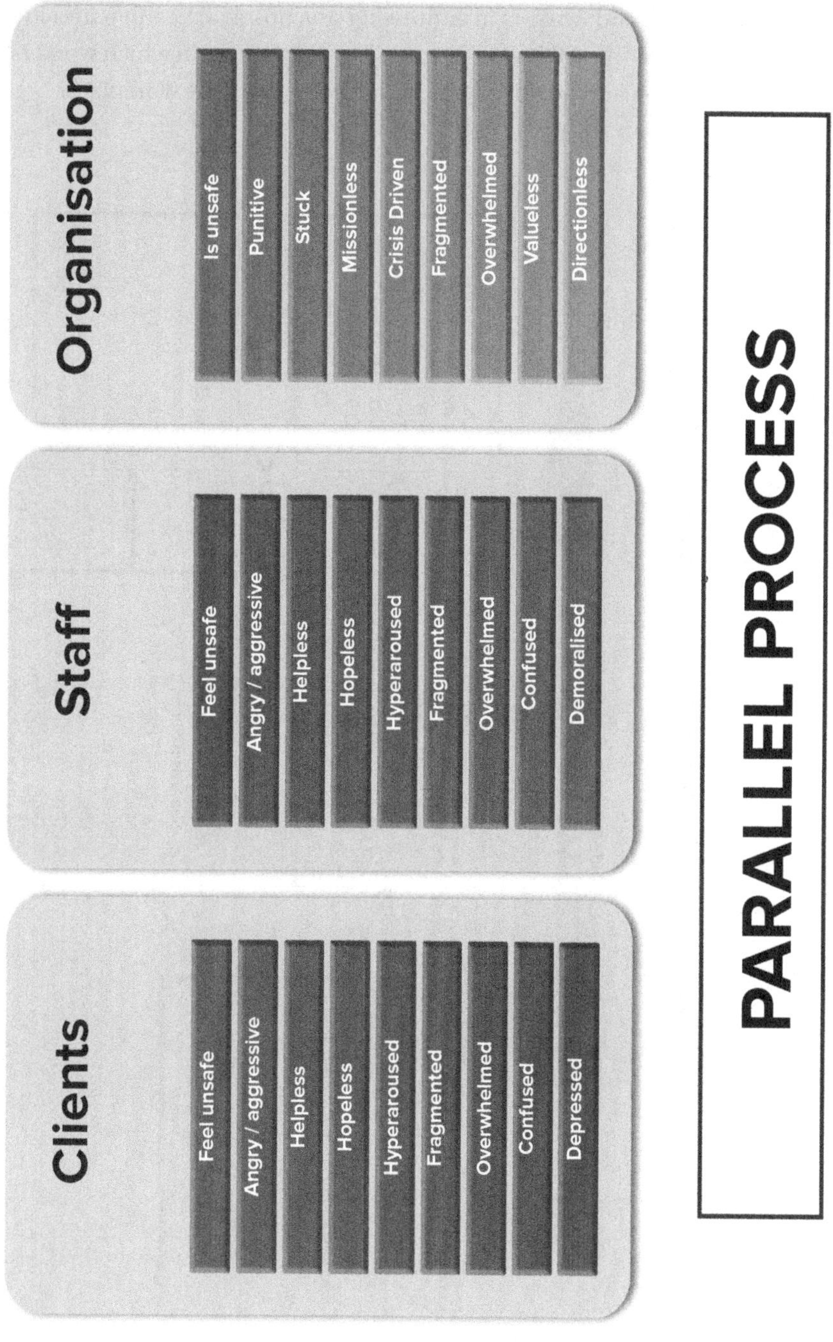

Psychosocial safety in the workplace

The Psychosocial Safety Climate Model has been developed to support managers and workers in addressing psychosocial health issues in the workplace. The following diagram highlights ways in which workers' motivation and health can be impacted upon in the workplace.

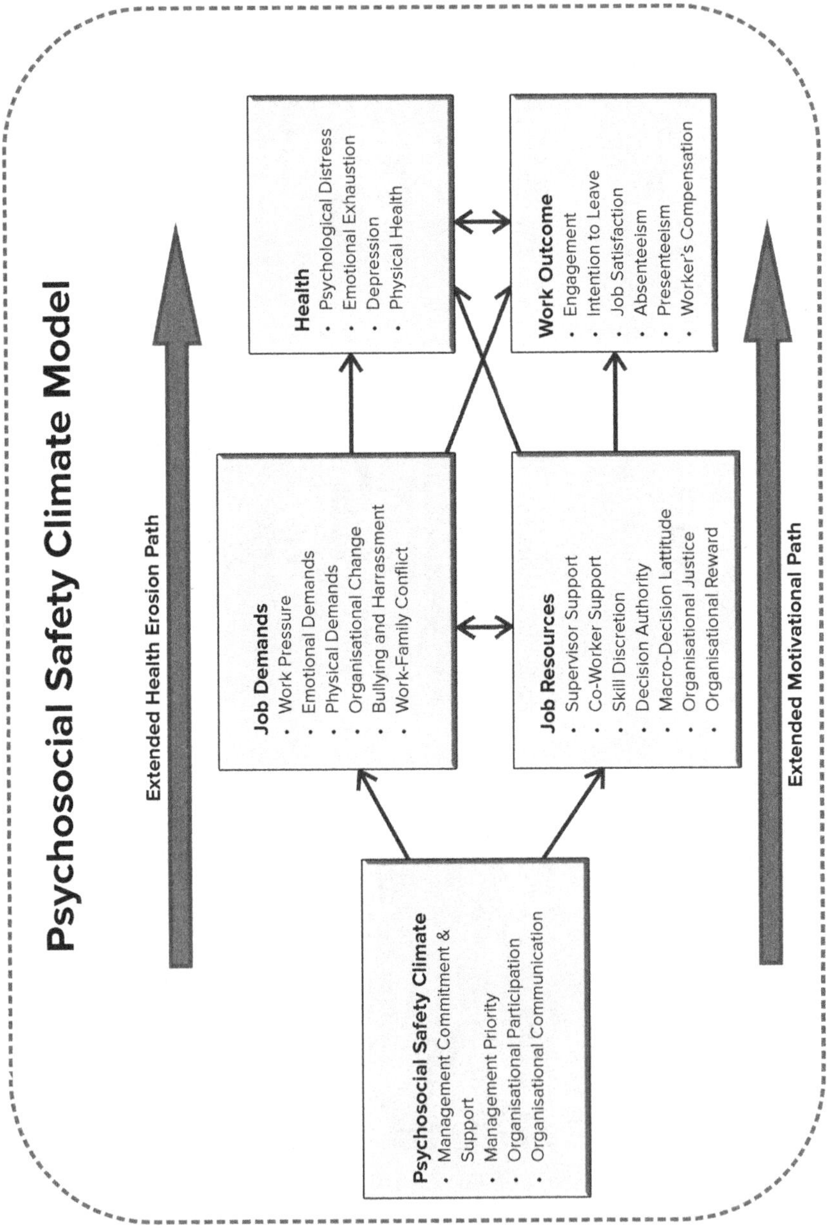

Work-family conflicts, work pressures, emotional demands, and bullying and harassment are recognised as having the most damaging effects on psychological health (Dollard, M. et al, page 40). There is no doubt at all that managers and their management style influence the effectiveness of trauma workers. For trauma workers who are trauma survivors in particular, aspects of the managerial style could inadvertently increase stress and trauma.

I once had the experience of working in a trauma organisation where the managers perceived themselves as highly fair and ethical. There were rules in the organisation about what people could and could not discuss with one another and there were 13 different ways that I could be told about the mistakes other people were making without the individual concerned knowing about it. There was little laughter in this organisation and it was once described to me as having a surveillance culture. You can imagine then that trauma workers in this organisation would become concerned about what they were doing and whether they were doing anything wrong. While this kept people on their toes, it was not conducive to building a team that trusted and supported one another. For trauma workers who were trauma survivors, their confidence could easily be eroded. They were inadvertently encouraged to tell on one another so that measures could be implemented to 'correct' behavior and attitudes. Just surviving in this type of organisation led to experienced staff leaving after a short time and, since the managers blamed those who were leaving as 'not being able to survive the work like they had', there was little opposition to the oppressive culture they had built and the high organisational and financial costs in the constant round of searching for and recruiting new staff continued to mount.

In another organisation providing support services to people who had experienced a traumatic illness, the manager would play his senior staff off against one another by publically congratulating specific senior staff in a manner to increase competitiveness amongst them. This organisation had around 90% staff turnover every 12 months. The board who managed the organisation with donations and public moneys rarely queried what must be happening in the organisation for such a high staff turnover to occur. Neither did they respond when they discovered that the CEO's private business website inferred the organisation was his client and not his employer.

It is not rocket science that the managers of any organisation will have a profound impact on people's experiences at work. I remember when one of my own employees who had been incarcerated and tortured in a foreign country remarked to me, *'you don't have to just be a good manager in trauma services, you also must be able to manage us when we are crazy not just from the work we do, but what we have also experienced.'* I felt at the time this was high praise indeed. However there are specific factors in the workplace that can potentially lead to vicarious trauma in staff. These include caseload sizes, the worker's personal trauma histories, and whether people feel they have the training they need for the work they do.

Some of the concerns I have observed amongst managers of trauma services is their lack of knowledge and understanding about how trauma affects the organisation. They are frequently employed in the non-government sector with limited clinical experience and are placed there by boards who may comprise faith based concerns or volunteers wanting to 'give their time' and rarely turning up to meetings due to their busy work lives and businesses. This often leaves trauma organisations in a kind of limbo. They try to meet the demands of people who have only worked in corporate organisations and who have limited understanding of the effects of trauma on workers. The organisational culture becomes focused on this corporatisation with limited understanding of human rights management. They make attempts to implement trauma-informed approaches through their staff which, while laudable, clients do need workers who understand trauma and its impacts and what is often overlooked is the review and evaluation of services from a trauma-informed perspective. In what ways, then, do such organisations policies, processes, and practices traumatise their own staff and clients?

Seven mistakes I have seen in the management of trauma services:

1. Taking the money no matter what

Many trauma services survive on non-renewable funding, or funding from different government and non-government departments. While I do not want to trivialise the legitimacy of this, I have seen some of these often smaller non-government organisations have different rules for different staff depending on funding cycles instead of managers negotiating with funding bodies about how the funding could be implemented in a core organisational policy context.

Sometimes it is necessary to refuse funds that cannot be woven into the organisational context rather than agreeing to funds tied to policies that do not support the cause.

2. 'We were the first service and are the experts so we know best'

Being pioneers in a trauma field is challenging and hard for both staff and managers involved. However I have seen managers and services become stagnant as they retain what they do, believing themselves to be the 'true' experts and discounting the contributions of other knowledges and perspectives. For example, in one small country I saw seven services develop in response to the main service's lack of collaboration with other services and views. What occurred was constant competition for the same funds and a discounting of one another's work. This resulted in clients becoming confused about which services were most suitable for them. While healthy debates increase knowledge in a field, ongoing 'turf' battles and competitiveness undermines the credibility of organisations and their service delivery. Building in an evaluation program to service development can assist organisations to manage change required by the external environment.

3. Human rights as rhetoric not substance

In one of the examples above where strict rules were in place about who staff could speak to, and what staff could speak about, many workers felt they were working in a surveillance environment, and shared the demoralising experience of their clients despite the organisation defining itself as a human rights organisation. While the mangers of this organisation believed they were maintaining a calm work environment providing, as they saw it, a 'containing context', it in fact had the opposite effect. Reviewing organisation policy against relevant human rights instruments can assist to address this mismatch.

4. Trauma-informed for clients — not staff

I have often reflected on my observation that many human rights and trauma related organisations implement systems for staff that go against the principles of being either trauma-informed or human rights advocating.

While studying at Harvard University's Frances Bignauld Centre for Health and Human Rights, we were encouraged to take a piece of policy or practice from our own country and systematically review this against the United Nations Declaration of Human Rights. The exercise was aimed at giving us clarity about what complied and also to consider what some of the reasons were when implementation was stymied. I recently set a similar task to a social work student working in a youth service. The student was able to link what he saw in the survey with international standards and it provided for him a context to the work beyond simply running recreational services.

In the same way, taking a client's view of our services is important – what is the client experience from first point of contact through their entire journey with our agency? Does the client know exactly what data we keep on them? Do they understand the reasons why we are referring them to someone else? Are there clear pathways clients have choices about? By the same token are there practices in the centre that staff experience as trauma-informed for them? I have observed how staff morale is undermined when they are belittled in public by managers or colleagues and little action is taken.

5. Long hours in the same role

There is evidence that vicarious trauma occurs when people are exposed to traumatic material in the workplace. However I have also seen work patterns in trauma organisations becoming crystallised. People are not provided variety in their work roles.

Other skills they have are not acknowledged and there are limited opportunities to use their creativity in their work. In one service I managed, every person in the organisation could work on a project they were passionate about which did not focus on the skills they used in their major role.

As the manager in that service I was able to participate in specific group work programs such as photography and storytelling projects which were important to the organisation and were not part of my day-to-day role. The criteria for the projects was that it was something they were passionate about doing which was not part of their normal work load and it further added to the work we were doing as an organisation.

6. Dignity has low priority

Consider the earlier example in one organisation where I could be provided with information about a specific staff member's non-compliance with policy through 13 different processes in the organisation.

While this was considered in the organisation as providing checks and balances, it tended to encourage information sharing about individual staff members across one layer in the organisation in such a way that the individual staff member had no knowledge of it nor could counteract it. When I raised this as an issue with a senior manager I was accused of *'auditing the managers.'*

It was disappointing that this lack of transparency with staff members was not seen as an issue that could negatively impact upon workers' dignity. I believe that how we dignify our staff as well as our clients influences the outcomes for our clients.

7. Gendered management

In organisational re-structures in trauma and human rights organisations I have often seen a lack of equity in management structures. For example, feminist organisations that refuse to employ men when significant numbers of their clientele are men. Human rights organisations employing men in senior roles and providing limited space for women. Non-government, not for profit organisations often had only a few women on their boards with limited opportunities for them to progress.

While this can be reflective of the wider community context in which organisations function, when managing trauma related organisations with a human rights perspective, it is important the whole organisation critically reflect on its own story and structure.

What can managers do?

- Share the story of how your organisation came into being
- Evaluate principles, policies and practices against relevant human rights and trauma-informed documentation
- Know what you will accept funding for and what you won't
- Build an evaluation culture into the organisation designed around quality indicators of practice and empowerment evaluation principles
- Develop processes enabling staff to clarify their own strategies for preventing vicarious trauma and burnout
- Review the structures of your teams

Chapter 16

An ending to a 'not quite' ending

I have not completed my career in trauma work. I consult with boards and managers of trauma organisations, supervise trauma clinicians, conduct training, and see clients with complex trauma histories. Dr Dimity Podger from Barasa Consulting group (an organisation that engages organisation leaders in values-based changes) asked me an interesting question: 'What is it that keeps people going through this kind of work?' I paused for a moment, took a breath and told her I could only reflect on what keeps *me* in this work.

It is my belief that trauma workers need the kind of valuing and respect and care that we give our clients. A lot is said in the current literature about being *'trauma-informed.'* While I value the concepts behind this approach that forces organisations to look closely at how their policies, systems and structures affect clients, I am not sure we have totally developed the policies, systems and structures that support those working with complex and difficult traumas in their work contexts.

Too often I have seen major health and mental health issues develop in trauma workers once they have left the field. It is as though all the giving to others leaves them worn-out, exhausted, with relationship challenges in their immediate families.

As more than one worker has said, *'it's working out what to do next when you have been involved in such meaningful work'* that can be so difficult. I have seen more than one family member desperate for the time when their partner, son, daughter, or parent puts as much commitment into their family as they have done with their clients.

Arianna Huffington in her book *'Thrive: The Third Metric to Redefining Success and Creating a Life of Well-Being, Wisdom, and Wonder'* argues effectively for the importance of building more into our lives that can sustain us beyond the life's work we do. I developed the following infographic from her book as a summary of key practices which trauma workers can build into their day-to-day lives where their investment is on the day-to-day meaningful relationships with themselves, those close to them, and those they just share moments and space with. As the slow food movement has revolutionised the way people buy and prepare food for themselves and their families, these thrive-practices reorient us to how to be in our own moments rather than in someone else's trauma stories or in our own.

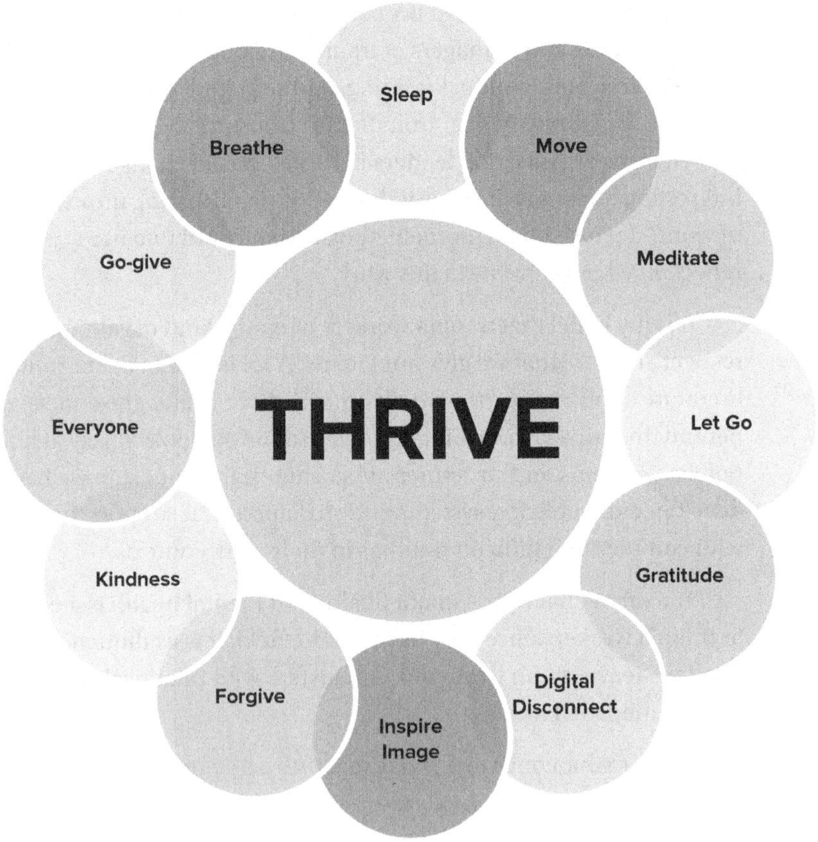

I began this book with a story of my sitting with my friend as she was diagnosed with cancer. During the writing of this book she died peacefully never giving up hope for a miracle. After 10 years my daughter has made contact — by email at this stage. She is married and is happy and I have a grandson — my fourth grandchild. Our lives as trauma workers evolve and change and, like our clients, we too face challenges in the cycles of our own living. And in the materiality of our own life all we can do is our best.

And one more thought:

Caretake this moment.

Immerse yourself in particulars.

Respond to this person, this challenge, this deed.

As concerns the art of living,

the material is your own life.

No great thing is created suddenly.

There must be time.

Give your best and

always be kind.

(Epictetus)

BIBLIOGRAPHY

American Psychiatric Association (2013) 'Diagnostic and Statistical Manual of Mental Disorders, (5th ed.).' Washington, DC: Author

Bloom, S. and B. Farragher (2010) 'Destroying Sanctuary: The Crisis in Human Service Delivery Systems.' Oxford: Oxford University Press

Boss, P. (2006) 'Loss, Trauma, and Resilience Therapeutic Work with Ambiguous Loss.' New York: Norton

Dollard, M., T. Bailey, S. McLinton, P. Richards, W. McTernan, A. Taylor and S. Bond (2012) 'Australian Workplace Barometer Report on Psychosocial Safety Climate and Worker Health in Australia.' Sydney: Safe Work Australia

Fedler, Joanne (2008) 'Things without a Name.' Sydney: Allen and Unwin

Felitti, V.J., R.F. Anda, D. Nordenberg, D.F. Williamson, A.M. Spitz, V. Edwards, M.P. Koss and J.S. Marks (1998) 'Relationship of childhood abuse and household dysfunction to many of the leading causes of death in adults. The Adverse Childhood Experiences (ACE) Study.' *American Journal of Preventitive Medicine* 14(4): 245–58

Frankl, Victor (2004) 'Man's Search for Meaning.' London: Rider and Co

Herman, Judith (1992) 'Trauma and Recovery: The Aftermath of Violence from Domestic Abuse to Political Terror.' New York: Basic Books

Huffington, Arianna (2014) 'Thrive: The Third Metric to Redefining Success and Creating a Life of Well-Being, Wisdom, and Wonder.' London: WH Allen

Hudgins, K. (2002) 'Experiential Treatment of PTSD: The Therapeutic Spiral Model.' New York: Springer Publishing Co

Levine, Peter A. (2008) 'Healing Trauma: A Pioneering Program for Restoring the Wisdom of Your Body.' Louisville, CO: Sounds True

Pert, Candice (1999) 'Molecules of Emotion: The Science Behind Mind-Body Medicine.' New York: Scribner

Quotes - http://www.brainyquote.com

Richardson, Cheryl (2002) 'Life Makeovers: 52 Practical and Inspiring Ways to Improve your Life One Week at a Time.' New York: Broadway Books

Siebert, A. (2010) 'The Survivor Personality.' New York: Perigee Books

Smith, K.K., V.M. Simmons and T.B. Thames (1989) '"Fix the Women": An Intervention into an Organizational Conflict Based on Parallel Process Thinking.' *The Journal of Applied Behavioural Science* 25(1): 11–29

Snyder, C. R. (1994) 'The Psychology of Hope: You can get there from here.' New York: Free Press.

Snyder, C. R. (2002) 'Hope theory: Rainbows in the Mind.' *Psychological Inquiry* 13: 249–275

Zoellner, L.A. and N.C. Feeny (2014) 'Facilitating Resilience and Recovery Following Trauma.' London: Guildford Press

Made in the USA
Monee, IL
04 November 2026

67377030R00075